Combining Touch AND Relaxation Skills FOR Cancer Care

by the same author

Aromatherapy, Massage and Relaxation in Cancer Care
An Integrative Resource for Practitioners
Edited by Ann Carter and Dr Peter A. Mackereth
ISBN 978 1 84819 281 2
eISBN 978 0 85701 228 9

of related interest

Hand Reflexology for Practitioners
Reflex Areas, Conditions and Treatments
Nicola Hall
Foreword by Matthew Williams
ISBN 978 1 84819 280 5
eISBN 978 0 85701 227 2

Seven Scents
Healing and the Aromatic Imagination
Dorothy P. Abram
Illustrated by Laura Mernoff
ISBN 978 1 84819 349 9
eISBN 978 0 85701 307 1

Health, the Individual, and Integrated Medicine
Revisiting an Aesthetic of Health Care
David Aldridge
ISBN 978 1 84310 232 8
eISBN 978 1 84642 644 5

Aromatica
A Clinical Guide to Essential Oil Therapeutics
Peter Holmes LAc, MH
ISBN 978 1 84819 303 1
eISBN 978 0 85701 257 9

Aromatherapeutic Blending
Essential Oils in Synergy
Jennifer Peace Rhind
ISBN 978 1 84819 227 0
eISBN 978 0 85701 174 9

Comforting Touch in Dementia and End of Life Care
Take My Hand
Barbara Goldschmidt and Niamh van Meines
Illustrated by James Goldschmidt
ISBN 978 1 84819 073 3
eISBN 978 0 85701 048 3

Combining Touch AND Relaxation Skills FOR Cancer Care

The HEARTS Process

Ann Carter
Assistant Author: Peter A. Mackereth

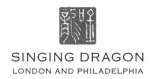

SINGING DRAGON
LONDON AND PHILADELPHIA

First published in 2019
by Singing Dragon
an imprint of Jessica Kingsley Publishers
73 Collier Street
London N1 9BE, UK
and
400 Market Street, Suite 400
Philadelphia, PA 19106, USA

www.singingdragon.com

Library of Congress Cataloging in Publication Data
A CIP catalog record for this book is available from the Library of Congress

British Library Cataloguing in Publication Data
A CIP catalogue record for this book is available from the British Library

ISBN 978 1 84819 352 9
eISBN 978 0 85701 311 8

Printed and bound by CPI Group (UK) Ltd, Croydon, CR0 4YY

This book is dedicated to all the patients and carers who have experienced the HEARTS Process and to the therapists, healthcare professionals and care workers who are practising HEARTS. It is through their ongoing feedback and commitment that HEARTS has grown into the effective therapeutic process that is being practised today.

CONTENTS

DISCLAIMER

Complementary therapy practices are constantly evolving in response to research, service evaluations, the needs of patients (and carers) and concurrent developments in medical practice. It is the responsibility of the therapist to maintain professional development and to work within the policies and practices of the context of his/her own clinical and private practice. The contributors and publisher are not responsible for any harm or damage to a person, no matter how caused as a result of information shared in this book.

ACKNOWLEDGEMENTS

First, I would like to thank Dr Peter Mackereth for his invaluable help in the writing of this book. Without Peter's assistance, it would have been difficult to complete the text, and I am grateful for his expertise, commitment and support in bringing the book to a successful conclusion.

My thanks also go to Salma Chaudhry, Jenny Gilbert, Ann Marie McGrath, Hassan Pillai and Christine Uphill for writing about their experiences of HEARTS to 'set the scene', providing insights into the practice of HEARTS in cancer care.

Next, I would like to thank my friends and colleagues for their knowledge and expertise in commenting on the draft texts and suggesting resources for inclusion. I also appreciate their support and interest in the book, which has been continuous since the start of the project. They are Joanne Barber, Anne Cawthorn, Tim Jackson, Fokkina McDonnell, Paula Maycock, Anita Mehrez, Lynne Tomlinson and Jan Williams. Additionally, many thanks to Marianne Tavares, who set up the interview with me that formed the framework for Chapter 1.

Thank you to Adele Kinsella of the Lifesong Project who sent me examples of many situations where HEARTS has been practised in care and nursing homes in the North East of England. This material offered valuable insights into using HEARTS with older people, which were integrated into Chapter 10.

I would like to thank Fiona James and acknowledge her artistic skills in producing the drawing of the Homunculus in Chapter 3. Thanks must also go to all the therapists who took part in an impromptu 'photo shoot' on a recent HEARTS course, as well as everyone who contributed to the photographs.

One of the principle features of the book is the summary of the questionnaire results in Chapter 12. Thank you to all the therapists who returned the questionnaire and for sending me so many heart-warming case histories about the practice of HEARTS.

And finally, Peter and I would like to thank Denise Rankin Box, Dr Jacqui Stringer and Jonathan Benavides for their endorsements of the book. Their professional comments are much appreciated by both of us.

PREFACE:
THE HEARTS PROCESS

Welcome to this book about the practice of the HEARTS Process. For some readers, this book may be your first introduction to HEARTS, so I thought you may like to know of other therapists' experience of using the approach, setting the scene for your own exploration of this book.

Ann Marie McGrath, Complementary therapist and HEARTS teacher, Dublin, Ireland

As a complementary therapist working in hospice care for over 16 years, I have found the HEARTS Process provides more options for approaching complementary therapy sessions with clients. The HEARTS techniques are gentle, and comfort-orientated, and can be tailored to meet the needs of individuals with complex medical conditions and who are often quite frail. Often, patients wish their close family members/loved ones to stay with them as much as possible. This provides an opportunity to teach them how they can apply some of the HEARTS techniques, to give some comfort to their loved one. The HEARTS Process blends well with the philosophy of palliative care in providing comfort care to individuals with life-limiting illness, right up to the end of life.

Christine Uphill, Complementary therapist and HEARTS teacher, Harrogate, Yorkshire, England

After practising HEARTS for six years I continue to be astounded at the positive outcomes I see for patients and carers. It is not just the versatility and rapid results that are so amazing with HEARTS. I use HEARTS for patients who are too ill to remove clothing for a treatment, and for their stressed-out friends and family. Often, patients and their carers are completely exhausted, and the gentle, 'nurturing' touch of HEARTS seems to transport them back to a time when they were worry-free and safe, bringing a sense of relief and peace!

Hassan Pillai, Complementary therapist and trustee, Macclesfield Cancer Help Centre, Cheshire, England

It is so beautiful when you see, and feel, the peace that follows, when anxiety, which is also grief, is washed away with a caring and soothing touch. HEARTS introduced me to that rounded and intimate approach, which opens doors for the giver and receiver, while it is also so easy to evaluate. I have used HEARTS in a cancer support environment, engaging partners/relatives, all feeling empowered to release emotions. Beautiful and healing.

Jenny Gilbert, Complementary therapist and HEARTS teacher, Stirling, Scotland

My practice as a therapist working with cancer and palliative care patients changed completely after attending the HEARTS Process workshop many years ago, as it encouraged me to work more intuitively with patients. Patients and carers have reported feelings of amazement that they can feel so relaxed, nurtured, loved and peaceful with such gentle, empathic touch over a blanket – what greater gift can one human being give to another?

Salma Chaudhry, Complementary therapist specialising in cancer care, Manchester, England

I work in an oncology setting and I feel very privileged to have learned the HEARTS Process, which I have used for the last five years. Due to the complexities of some patients' conditions, there may be limitations as to how we use our therapies even though we have learned to adapt and integrate them. With HEARTS there is complete gentleness, and now I never need to say 'no' to a patient.

One of the beauties of HEARTS is its blend of ingredients which enables a synergy between the warmth of the hands and the stillness they create. Together, they infuse a sense of relaxation that flows through the body, creating a sense of peace which acts almost as an invitation to the patient to let go of any anxieties.

HEARTS has enhanced my toolbox, but more importantly, it has enriched the patient's sense of self.

INTRODUCTION AND
OVERVIEW OF THE BOOK

But O for the touch of a vanish'd hand,
And the sound of a voice that is still!

> Extract from the poem 'Break, Break, Break' by Alfred, Lord
> Tennyson (1842, quoted in Autton 1989, p.108)

HEARTS is an acronym that encompasses a group of therapeutic approaches: Hands-on, Empathy, Aromas, Relaxation, Textures and Sound. The essence of HEARTS is simplicity, and the intention is for the process to be accessible to anyone, at any time, and in any place. Of course, the giving and receiving of HEARTS depends on continuing consent, with most treatments lasting for between 5 and 20 minutes. The recipient does not need to remove clothing and treatments are tailored to meet the needs of individual patients and carers.

All HEARTS treatments involve the use of touch through the Hands-on work that is delivered either through the textures of clothing or through an additional fabric cover. Sometimes, patients benefit from something 'extra' to the sense of touch through the use of Sound to promote feelings of calm and relaxation. This is offered through simple relaxation techniques using the sound of the human voice (and/or music, if this is available). The final sense we use in HEARTS is the sense of smell (Aromas). This can be offered through individual person-centred guided imagery (PCGI), the use of essential oils or through reference to familiar aromas. All these approaches can also be integrated into complementary treatments, such as massage, aromatherapy and reflexology.

Although HEARTS is often used in supportive and palliative situations, it is suitable for patients and carers at any stage of the cancer journey and also for our colleagues, friends and families. The techniques have also been used in many other situations such as care and nursing homes, for people with Down's syndrome and multiple sclerosis, and wherever there has been a need for a brief, effective technique that can help an individual to calm and access a more balanced state of wellbeing.

Composite case histories have been included in this book that illustrate the principles discussed and the outcomes of treatments. All chapters begin with keywords and a short introduction. At the end of each chapter is a summary, and recommendations for good practice are included either at the end of the chapter or throughout the text.

HEARTS has been described as 'a hug in a rug, a pleasure to give and a joy to receive'. I hope that the techniques described will be transferable to other areas of your work.

Part 1 is concerned with the fundamentals of HEARTS. Chapter 1 looks at the history of HEARTS and the logic that has supported its development. Chapter 2 is about the sense of touch, reviewing the role that this often 'under-rated' sense plays in our everyday lives. In HEARTS, the skin is referred to metaphorically as the 'canvas on which we paint our art', so in Chapter 3, the structure of the skin and the skilful use of hands are considered in relationship to the sensory system and its integral connection with the brain.

Part 2 is concerned with the six components of HEARTS. These are not approached in the order of the acronym, but are presented in what seemed to be a more logical order for the readers' benefit. Chapter 4 explores the concept of empathy that underpins all therapeutic interactions. It is an essential component of every HEARTS treatment, both in the verbal interactions with the patient or carer, and in using empathy with the hands. This chapter also includes a discussion about the nature of empathy, compassion and sympathy, with some techniques for developing empathy, and suggestions for remaining grounded and not becoming over-involved. Chapter 5 focuses on the relaxation process, providing suggestions and recommendations for good practice. The chapter concludes with a review of some research papers related to guided imagery.

Chapters 6, 7 and 8 cover the three components of HEARTS that involve practical skills. Chapter 6 includes the benefits of working through textures and gives details of the Library of Strokes and some of the differences between HEARTS and massage. Chapter 7 covers the therapeutic use of sound. In the context of HEARTS, sound is either the skilful use of music or the use of your own voice (or a combination of both). PCGI approaches are recommended for use as far as possible, and where appropriate. Some suggestions are also included for integrating the use of the voice with the touch work, as ways of building confidence in this very useful area of HEARTS. Chapter 8 is then concerned with aromas, and offers two approaches. The first is to facilitate PCGI by asking the patient to recall or think of an aroma that suggests a narrative for the imagery. This method enables the use of aromas to be available to everyone. The second approach concerns the use of essential oils, which can only be prescribed by a qualified aromatherapist. Where appropriate, the two approaches can be coordinated.

Part 3 covers the role that HEARTS can play in the care of people who have cancer, for both the patients and their carers. Chapter 9 presents an overview of cancer, its treatments and a potential role for HEARTS. Examples of integrating HEARTS in patient care are described through case histories in a variety of situations. Recognising the increasing age of the population and the increasing incidence of dementia, memory loss and cancer among older people, Chapter 10 explores the use of HEARTS for this highly complex target group. The nature of dementia and memory loss in the context of cancer care is discussed, together with implications for carers and recommendations as to how therapists can work with patients who have memory loss or dementia. (These recommendations may also be helpful to therapists working with older people.)

Chapter 11 covers teaching and learning for two target groups. The first section of the chapter outlines the current arrangements for training therapists, healthcare professionals and healthcare workers to use HEARTS. These courses are open to anyone who has a role to play in supportive and palliative care settings, and in care and nursing homes. The second section covers how carers perceive HEARTS and its benefits, describing some characteristics of the carer as an adult learner and the effect that individual learning styles may have on the way in which carers respond.

Chapter 12 is the final chapter of the book, and describes the results of a questionnaire that was circulated to therapists who had completed the two days' training. This is the first time that an attempt has been made to gather some quantifiable data. The results are very positive and support the experiences that have been described since the creation of HEARTS in the mid-1990s. Therapists disclosed a variety of the problems they face, and some of these have been addressed in the book.

The Appendix contains a copy of the questionnaire, and this is followed by References, and finally Further Reading and Online Resources, providing a list of books that have inspired the development of the HEARTS Process together with some useful book resources and online sources.

Part 1

THE FOUNDATION
OF HEARTS

Chapter 1

THE STORY OF THE HEARTS PROCESS

Marianne Tavares interviews Ann Carter

Question 1. Why was there a need for HEARTS?

As a therapeutic intervention, HEARTS did not start out with a name of any kind; the name that is based on the acronym came later. When I started working at the Neil Cliffe Centre for cancer care in Manchester in 1992, it soon became clear that my training in massage and aromatherapy was not sufficiently flexible. For me to work effectively with people who had a life-threatening illness, my practice had to change to meet the needs of patients who had a wide variety of existing problems. From the onset of working in cancer care, I encountered difficulties; sometimes, for example, a patient's skin was very friable or resistant to absorbing a lubricant; the lubricant was typically grape seed oil, chosen for its ability to moisturise dry skin and facilitate a smooth glide during effleurage. For very poorly patients, positioning and creating comfort on a massage couch could be difficult. There were also body image issues, sometimes not verbally expressed, which surfaced when a patient was asked to remove even a minimal amount of clothing to receive a massage. Additionally, many patients, often those living with fatigue and the side effects of medication, were unable to accept a session that was scheduled to last an hour, although the hands-on work lasted only for a maximum of 40 minutes.

The day centre in which I was working as a complementary therapist was adjacent to a hospital ward. At that time, an oncology consultant who was linked with the day centre gave permission for therapists to work with in-patients when time was available. This amazing opportunity was an 'on the edge' experience, and it quickly became apparent that the treatment had to be adapted so it was acceptable to both the patient and the body posture of the therapist.

Treatments were usually offered to patients who were supported by pillows, and who were in either a seated or supine position. Therapists who were working in the centre needed to become familiar with the mechanics of hospital beds, and the need to remove bed ends for easier access to the patient. Additionally, there were complications of medical paraphernalia, such as intravenous lines, drainage catheters, oxygen masks and often-cluttered bed tables.

We needed to do something with our intention to help, using the complementary skills that we had. We all wanted to optimise this wonderful opportunity to make a difference to the wellbeing of vulnerable patients. Massage was not always appropriate, and neither was the use of essential oils. A gentle approach to reflexology was (and continues to be) very useful for patients as they do not need to disrobe and the feet are often easily accessible. However, for some patients, attention to the feet was not welcomed, and reflexology was not offered where there was local infection, altered sensation or where limbs were missing. Additionally, some patients requested attention to other areas of the body. The dilemma was to find a flexible approach that we could integrate safely and comfortably into our existing practice of complementary therapies. Whatever we did, the approach would need to meet the many challenges that arise when working in cancer care.

Question 2. So what influenced the development of HEARTS?

Possibly, the first major turning point was my visit to a Mind, Body, Spirit festival in London where I was helping on a stand sponsored by the (then) International Society of Professional Aromatherapists (ISPA). I was fascinated by how many of the therapies that were being demonstrated involved the skilful use of touch. The most significant therapies I noticed that involved kind, well-intentioned touch were shiatsu, the Metamorphic technique, Indian-style head massage and spiritual healing. (This doesn't mean to say that there weren't others, but these were the ones that had the most significance for me.) I noticed three things. First, members of the public who were receiving a short 'treatment' did not have to remove clothing. Second, amidst the loud noise of the crowds, and the continual variety of announcements over the speaker system, the giver and receiver of the therapy somehow created their own 'bubble of tranquillity'. This 'bubble' was obvious, although the giver and receiver were being observed by as many as 30 people. Third, the receiver was demonstrating signs of being in a relaxed state, despite being surrounded by observers. One woman, who was receiving Indian-style head massage, was so relaxed that she was visibly dribbling! In addition, she was leaning to one side of the chair, which had no arms, and I wondered if she would manage to remain seated! Potential distractions were overcome by what appeared to be a deepening 'connection' between the giver and receiver. Both parties were totally engaged; the giver was clearly absorbed in what s/he was doing and the receiver appeared to have willingly accepted the process.

For me, these three observable elements were important principles that triggered some reflective thoughts about my own touch-based practice. The massage I had learned required a lubricant that was applied to the receiver's skin. The approach was very much directed towards treating private clients, usually paying for one-hour sessions, or working in a gym or a beauty salon. As a trainee therapist, I had learned a set routine for the massage process, which formed the basis for the final practical assessment. However, in the hospice and cancer care context in which I was now working, I needed to revise and enhance my skill level. I felt it was important to make the best use of the time allocated, and to offer an effective and resourceful treatment for a patient or carer.

Question 3. How did these insights affect your evolving practice in cancer care?

When reviewing and revising my touch-based work, I took the principles I had learned at the festival and applied them to my work at the centre. First, a complementary therapy could be offered at the bedside in a busy ward environment and, in spite of the noise, relaxation and calm could still be achieved. We could create a therapeutic space around the bed. Second, if touch could be offered through fabric (clothes or covers) then patients would feel less exposed and less vulnerable. This would give us options which would create opportunities for patients with more complex needs. The third factor which influenced my practice was the versatility of touch techniques I had observed through watching a variety of approaches to body work. There were many ways in which skilful touch could be used which was not restricted to basic massage strokes.

Around this time I had been attending some short courses where gentle touch techniques were involved. I started adapting some of the techniques for use with clothed patients and was very pleased with the outcomes and the feedback. The 'adapted' techniques were empathic, gentle and effective, and it was these approaches that became central to the HEARTS Process.

In the first instance, I offered treatments using the touch techniques to some very vulnerable patients who were covered with large towels throughout the treatment. The responses from patients and their carers, who often sat in on the sessions, were positive and encouraging. So, with the permission of the oncology consultant and a GP who was also involved with the centre, I began integrating these approaches regularly within my practice.

Question 4. Why did you feel it necessary to introduce the use of sound?

As I provided more and more treatments using adapted touch techniques, it became clear to me that there was still a missing component. Most patients wanted to access a state of relaxation or at least a state of calm. Some patients had difficulty in achieving this state with touch therapies alone. The hands-on work was enjoyed and regarded as pleasurable, but for some patients it wasn't enough to calm the 'chattering thoughts'. I noticed that some patients wanted to chat throughout the whole treatment, or they would relax for a short while, and then start to chat again. Frequently, patients talked about having 'overactive and sometimes intrusive thoughts' so they weren't able to 'switch off'. It seemed easier for patients to disengage from the relaxation process, as they did not have a resourceful strategy for coping with internal chatter. I needed to add something that would engage their thoughts and offer an easily accessible solution. Music was an obvious option, but in some situations there was no access to a CD player, so another approach had to be devised. Some patients asked for a technique that they could learn and practise at home, so different methods had to be created that involved the patient in some way. If the patient was cognitively able, it would be something s/he could use to help 'self soothe' when a therapist was not present. (I describe these processes in detail in Chapter 7 on 'Sound'.)

As a result of practising a combination of well-intentioned touch and different methods to 'quieten the chattering mind', the patient's key healthcare workers at the hospice and cancer care centre asked me if I would give 'what I was doing' a name, so that patients could be referred specifically for this therapeutic package.

Question 5. How did you arrive at the name of 'HEARTS'?

One afternoon, the complementary therapy coordinator (who had been involved in the development of the approach) and myself sat down with flipchart paper and pens. Our aim was to devise a name for the collection of processes with which we had become very familiar. We isolated each component of the total approach and our first attempt produced the mnemonic 'HERTS' (Hands-on, Empathy, Relaxation, Textures and Sound). This was not a good title; no healthcare worker would want to refer a patient for an intervention by a name that suggests pain! It was at that point that we agreed to include aromatherapy, although we were aware that only qualified aromatherapists could prescribe essential oils. Since these early stages, 'Aromatherapy' has been modified to be included as 'Aromas', which gives all therapists using 'HEARTS' an additional therapeutic approach. The methods have been modified so that guided imagery involving aromas can be devised in a way that involves the patient. These are further described in Chapter 8.

Question 6. What has encouraged you to continue with the development of HEARTS?

There are many reasons. Principally, it was the benefits to the patients; it was like finding a 'missing link'. The feedback from the key workers and nurses about the effective outcomes for patients and carers was excellent, and the growing number of positive case histories was very heart warming. HEARTS was something that could be used almost anywhere, in any situation, and which could be effective in short periods of time. As a therapist, I also enjoyed using HEARTS in the challenging area of hospice and cancer care; I loved its flexibility and I came to regard HEARTS as an art form as well as one that had a scientific basis. The words that really offered inspiration and that I still quote at the start of every course I teach, are from Alfred, Lord Tennyson's poem, 'Break, Break, Break':

> But O for the touch of a vanish'd hand,
> And the sound of a voice that is still!

> (quoted in Autton 1989, p.108)

This is the essence of what HEARTS is all about.

Question 7. What response have you had from sharing and teaching HEARTS with complementary therapists?

Complementary therapists are always very keen to learn new skills that will enhance their practice and importantly support their patients. HEARTS has been greeted with enthusiasm on all of the courses. By the end of the workshops many of the therapists are thinking of patients for whom it would be suitable. Sometimes, I continue to meet therapists who were trained in the early days, which is now over 20 years ago. They are always keen to tell me that they are still using HEARTS, and how useful and effective it is.

Question 8. What evaluations have you done?

I think that most complementary therapists are aware of the need for evaluation, monitoring and audit. Much positive feedback has been obtained from listening to comments from patients, carers, complementary therapists and healthcare professionals. However, this feedback is informal and has a major qualitative element, and little has been done to obtain quantitative data. After a two-day course in HEARTS, I offer a HEARTS practitioner certificate. To complete the certificate, participants write up two case histories, which aim to demonstrate the competent use of different aspects of HEARTS. If the case histories demonstrate good reflective practice, a practitioner certificate is awarded. I always send the individual some feedback on their work and therapists are aware that the certificate is not a qualification; it is an acknowledgement that they are prepared to go further in the context of developing their skills in using HEARTS. There has been an enormous amount of useful information about the value and application of HEARTS in these case histories, and I hope therapists have also found my feedback helpful. In 2017, I circulated a questionnaire and the results are discussed in Chapter 12. The content gives some information about how therapists use HEARTS and their perceptions of its value to themselves, their patients and carers.

Question 9. In your experience, how has HEARTS helped patients in the earlier stages of palliative care?

I have found that patients and carers have benefited from HEARTS at all stages of cancer. Sometimes there is a misconception that HEARTS is only for patients with advanced illness and end of life, whereas it is suitable for patients and carers at any stage of the cancer journey.

Its main advantages for patients who are receiving palliative care are:

- Patients don't need to remove clothing, so it can be practised in a variety of situations.

- There is no lubricant, set techniques or routines. Once the basic principles have been learned, HEARTS is largely intuitive and carers find this helpful.

- Treatments can last for around 5 minutes as a minimum; it doesn't take long for HEARTS to be 'quietly effective'.

- HEARTS can be incorporated into other complementary therapies at any stage of the treatment.

- HEARTS can also be used in conjunction with medical treatments and clinical procedures.

- In some situations, HEARTS has been used to restore physical contact between family members where this interaction has lessened, or been limited, through illness and disability.

- HEARTS is easy to learn – the approach and pressure used are no more than we would use for stroking a baby, a cat or a dog. It is a very gentle and rhythmic therapeutic approach.

Question 10. How can families benefit from HEARTS at end of life?

Healthcare staff and families will often look forward to the patient's treatment with a complementary therapist; they appreciate the benefits that can be experienced through receiving a touch-based therapy. However, a therapist may not be available when required, such as during the night, or when a patient is distressed or unable to sleep. It is in these situations where HEARTS comes into its own; the process gives the family options and something in which they, too, can be involved.

One of the features of HEARTS is that there is an option for two therapists (or two people) to work simultaneously with a patient. A carer (or carers) can easily learn some hands-on approaches that can be offered when a therapist isn't present. The easiest way for a carer to learn some HEARTS approaches is for him/her to work alongside a therapist. Observing, then copying, how a therapist is working can lead to building confidence and any safety aspects can be discussed. Providing the patient is well enough, some approaches from HEARTS can be given to the carer in return. This may be a welcome option. Sometimes a patient feels that s/he is receiving 'all the attention' and their loved ones are 'missing out'. Being able to offer 'reciprocal' touch may help to restore relationships as the patient feels that the receiving of care is not all in one direction.

Many carers have reported how HEARTS has helped them to feel that they could do something for their family member or friend in the last hours of life. They have also described an opportunity to create a resourceful, lasting memory where the family was involved in saying farewell to a loved one.

Question 11. What is the future for HEARTS?

I would like to see HEARTS more widely used in a variety of healthcare settings, so I am training experienced therapists to run HEARTS courses in different parts of the country. I don't see HEARTS as another 'complementary therapy' – there is no professional body, no final exams and no assessments. I see HEARTS as being a therapeutic process that can be integrated into patient care. Some of the case histories in the book will illustrate its versatility and effectiveness…and will help to capture the essence of HEARTS and its potential uses.

Ideally, I would like there to be more criteria for entry into teacher training. At present, I know personally the therapists who want to do the training course. I remain in touch with them and the ones who are able to run HEARTS courses are meeting the challenges with professionalism and enthusiasm – and they are enjoying the teaching, which is really important.

Question 12. Is there anything else you would like to add?

This feels like a 'post script' or an 'epilogue'. Through writing this book I have come to realise two principles. First, although HEARTS is a pleasure to demonstrate and learn, the anatomy and physiology that brings about the positive outcomes is very complex. Even more surprising is that the nervous system could be processing the sensations of touch, the sound of music (or the human voice) and aromatic sensations all at the same time! This is amazing physiology and we take it for granted. Second, from all the case histories, the existing evidence base and the HEARTS questionnaire results, I believe that we totally under-estimate the inherent properties of body and mind to make a positive change of some kind. This potential is always there, no matter how ill or troubled someone might be. We just need to find the right key to help unlock this potential for an individual. So many therapists, healthcare professionals, familial carers and caregivers have found HEARTS to be an inspiration and a resource in promoting a positive quality of life. I hope that this book will provide both an inspiration and a resource for its readers.

Chapter 2

THE ROLE OF TOUCH IN EVERYDAY LIFE

KEYWORDS

touch; benefits of touch; fear of touch; touch history; touch hunger; oxytocin; sensory language; metaphors

INTRODUCTION

Touch is a biological and social phenomenon that exists in all human cultures and across the animal world. Every day we experience touch in many different interactions and situations, sometimes without realising it. In spite of its importance in our lives, however, we often take our sense of touch for granted.

This chapter provides a brief overview of the role that touch plays in Western society. The concept of a 'touch history' is considered, together with the ongoing need for touch as part of the human condition. The contribution that kind, well-intentioned touch can make to positive health is discussed, although not all touch is welcome, and the deleterious effects of intrusive touch are also explored. Comforting contact with pets and the production of oxytocin are described in the context of 'self-soothing'. Reference is made to the role that healthcare professionals can have in the way they use touch in the course of their everyday work. The chapter concludes with an overview of the role that sensory language and metaphors of touch play in the English language, although no physical contact has taken place. The chapter begins and concludes with a case study that illustrates the power of human touch in the simplest of caring actions.

Case study 2.1. Ethel's story

Ethel was 84. She lived alone and had a grown-up family who were living some distance away, so she was rarely able to see them. Weekly, she would visit a centre where her care needs were attended to, such as bathing, hairdressing and being able to socialise with people in her age group. On this occasion, two of the carers gave Ethel a bath and instead of 'giving her a wash', they gave a soapy back massage, using their hands and a big soapy sponge. To their surprise, Ethel started to doze, so the bath was emptied and Ethel was wrapped up in a big towel and supported until she returned to full wakefulness. When she opened her eyes, her first words were, 'Oh my, I've waited 80 years for that!'

So what might have been Ethel's experience of touch during her lifetime? Eighty years is a long time to wait for touch that is perceived as caring, unconditional and comforting. We all have a 'touch history' that represents our experience of touch from birth until the age we are now. Although each person's history will be unique, there are some experiences that we may have in common.

AN OVERVIEW OF TOUCH IN WESTERN SOCIETY

Sensitivity to touch begins when the baby is in the womb, particularly in the third trimester (Marx and Nagy 2017). It is likely that the first sensory experience of the newborn baby is through touch, provided initially by a midwife, a doula, or a close family member, before the baby has first contact with the mother. Bonding takes place with the use of loving, caring touch given through holding and cuddling, the baby often being wrapped in a soft fabric. It is an accepted premise that babies and infants who do not receive appropriate touch fail to thrive. Leboyer (1976) acknowledged that touch is vital to the development of the infant. He describes the importance of touch by asserting that that touch and massage are 'food' for the child, and are as essential as proteins, vitamins and minerals.

During the first six months of life, the stimulation through touch that babies experience could be described as 'affectionate' touch – babies are cuddled, stroked, rocked, carried, kissed and held. Other kinds of touch, such as 'instrumental touch', are used when a baby is being changed, bathed or dressed, or when the baby's limbs are being played with and gently moved. During the next six months of age, when babies start to crawl, observational studies have found that touch behaviours change (Ferber, Feldman and Makhoul 2008). Researchers observed that, at this age, the infants had greater access to a variety of objects. The maternal affectionate touch that was given in the first six months declined significantly, and the new kind of touch experienced by infants was more interactive, helping to accommodate this curiosity-centred mode of activity. Dyadic reciprocity between mother and infant increased and was preceded by affectionate touch only. Perhaps paternal touch is more complex, with social and cultural variants and expectations, as some fathers have less involvement in childcare, such as nappy changing and bathing. The new 'nurturing father' heralded in the latter years of the 20th century remains a poorly studied area. Although the traditional role of the father being an 'authority figure' may continue to influence new fathers, some will want more involvement in the care of their children (Guzzo 2011). There has been a call to promote baby massage by fathers, with evidence to suggest an increase in bonding and parental involvement in childcare (Cheng, Volk and Marini 2011; Mackereth 2003).

As children grow up, touching with parents tends to become less frequent and with reduced intimacy. Touch may still be used to show affection – in hand holding, kissing and hugging in fun games such as 'rough and tumble' – or in everyday activities, such as helping younger children to wash, dress and undress. Sometimes touch is used as punishment, and in more extreme situations, touch is instrumental in abuse. Additionally, there are situations where touch is in short supply. Settle (1991) describes her experience observing in a Romanian orphanage. The children were rarely touched and often 'winced' when they were first touched by massage therapists.

During adolescence, touch from an individual's peer group becomes more important, and familial touch may not be particularly welcome, especially when members of the peer group are present. However, there remains a need for closeness, physical contact and intimacy. During adolescence, touching by a parent may be linked to being treated as 'a child', or it may trigger embarrassment about a young person's changing body. Physical contact can also be associated with growing sexual awareness and experimentation.

Classic research by Argyle (1975) recognised that there are socially defined circumstances in adult life where touching is deemed acceptable. He suggests that touch plays a role during sexual activities with one's partner and in the casual circumstances of everyday life. These may include interactions with children and in various greetings and farewells with friends and family members. Touch has an important role to play at many celebrations and rituals, such as graduations, weddings, christenings, anniversaries and funerals. There are also rituals for touching in some team sports that are acceptable on the sports field, for example, in football. When a goal is scored, there are euphoric celebrations that involve touch. If some of the reactions were to be performed on the high street, or in other social situations, the response would probably be greeted with surprise, and possibly disapproval. However, in the context of 'the match', such demonstrations of euphoria seem to be quite acceptable and even to be expected.

As we get older, receiving touch declines, although the need for it probably remains. As we are living longer, we may find that families and friends, with whom touch was acceptable, may have moved away or perhaps died. This can lead to social isolation, which can have its own deleterious effects on health. Other groups who possibly receive the least positive touch in society include older people, prisoners in isolation, people who are homeless and where individuals have infections or disfigurements.

The role of touch will vary in different cultures, and given the multicultural nature of UK society, it may be helpful for therapists to undertake further reading about this fascinating subject.

TOUCH HUNGER

The skin is a sensory organ that is designed to receive touch (see Chapter 3). Humans have a need for touch, both physiologically and emotionally. Where there is a shortage of kind, well-intentioned touch, a phenomenon known as 'touch hunger' may result. Nelson (2007) suggests that babies who receive minimal touching from their caregivers can experience delays in later cognitive development, which may last for many years. Orphans who had been deprived of touch in some Eastern European institutions displayed impaired growth and cognitive development, as well as an elevated incidence of serious infections and attachment disorders (Frank *et al.* 1996). However, there are many situations where individuals are consciously aware that they need the touch of another human being. This may take the form of a hug, a cuddle, a hand to hold or just someone to be close to, even if the person is a relative stranger or is not well known to the individual. O'Neil and Calhoun (1975) studied a group of 42 people aged over 70 who were resident in a nursing home. They found that 'sensory deficits' and 'senile traits' such as irritability, forgetfulness, careless grooming or eating habits were present in residents who were not frequently touched. Residents who received touch, either given through massage, frequent stroking, hugs, squeezing of the hands and arms, together with affectionate touching of the head, showed fewer signs of senility and were more alert and better humoured than residents who were not frequently touched (see Chapter 10).

There is another side to touch hunger – the situation where children are not receiving kind touch when they may need it. Field *et al.* (1994) describe how children in a nursery school were touched very little, especially as the children grew up. In the data collected by Field and her team, the nursery staff reported that touching was rare because of their concerns that touch might be construed as sexual abuse. Subrahmanyam and Greenfield (2008) also suggest that with the increased use of mobile phones for communicating with peers, adolescents are missing out on physical contact, which plays an important role in teenage relationships.

THE ROLE OF OXYTOCIN

Oxytocin is a hormone produced by the hypothalamus. It plays a role in kissing, pregnancy, childbirth and bonding with a baby. It is also known as the 'cuddle hormone' or the 'love hormone' as it is released when people hug, snuggle up or bond socially. Touch that is well received by an individual increases the production of oxytocin and reduces the production of cortisol, which is one of the principle causes of stress and depression (see Chapter 5).

Morhenn, Beavin and Zak (2012) conducted a survey that involved 95 participants in a Californian hospital. The research team drew blood samples from all participants. After the blood draw, the control group ($n=30$) rested quietly for 15 minutes. Participants in the massage group ($n=65$) received 15 minutes of moderate pressure massage of the upper back. A second blood draw followed for both groups. In the massage group, there was a significant increase in the production of oxytocin and a significant decrease in cortisol when compared with the control group.

Oxytocin can also be produced in interactions between dogs and humans. Humans produce oxytocin when stroking or patting a dog, and oxytocin production also occurs in the dog, even when the animal is not being touched.

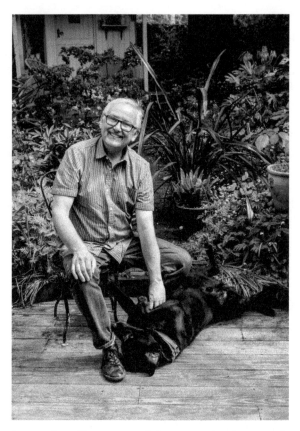

Figure 2.1. Humans and dogs can simultaneously
produce oxytocin for the enjoyment of both

Following a survey of research into the benefits of pets for senior citizens, Jorgenson (1996) reports on the benefits of keeping pets for this older age group. Senior citizens were found to have less cardiovascular illness and lived longer than those who did not have pets. It is possible that having physical contact through stroking and patting the animals, together with the sensory experience of the softness of the animal's fur, has replaced touch, which, at one time, was present in families or between friends. Stroking a pet may also be regarded as a method of self-help and may contribute to the process of self-soothing.

Increasingly, pets are also being used in supportive care situations such as care homes and hospices, with dogs (and cats) resident in some establishments. Alternatively, animals with a suitable temperament are brought into the care situation at appropriate times during the week. To help meet the needs of people in care, pets are increasingly being used to support people through fulfilling a person's needs to be touched and to give touch.

SELF-SOOTHING (SOMETIMES CALLED SELF-CALMING OR SELF-COMFORTING)

The *Concise Oxford English Dictionary* (2006) describes 'self-soothing' as 'to gently calm oneself'. An early stage of self-soothing for babies is for them to learn how to self-calm from crying to enter a state of quiet wakefulness, without parental intervention (Burnham *et al.* 2002). Self-soothing is a process that babies learn through sucking their thumbs or a comforter (dummy), or through having close contact with a favourite blanket or toy; the latter is likely to be soft and cuddly. Swaddling and carrying a child on the chest in a papoose have been advocated as a means of providing a continuing sense of comfort, as there is also some stimulation of the skin (Nelson 2017). As we go through childhood and adolescence on the way to becoming an adult, it is likely that we will learn strategies for calming ourselves that we can use in a variety of situations where we are anxious, fearful, angry or frustrated… We can learn to 'calm down', so we can cope with a difficult situation, or just promote a sense of wellbeing. Having a warm/hot bath with some pleasant aromas or bubbles can be a very relaxing experience. Making a warm drink is often used as a way to self-soothe, and in some contexts this simple action would enable the individual to 'have some space' and to 'chill' (see Chapter 5). There are other ways of self-soothing that involve the other senses of sight, sound, smell and taste. Some are less resourceful than others, such as smoking, high alcohol consumption and over-eating, but in the short term they may have the effect of helping the individual to feel better.

Physical warmth can also play an important role in self soothing. We may like to wrap ourselves in a soft dressing gown, cover ourselves with a blanket and sit somewhere that is warm and cosy. The textures and sensations of soft fabric may be helpful for individuals who receive very little touch. Although there is nothing that comes close to the feeling of kind touch from a human hand, wrapping oneself in a warm, soft blanket may subconsciously bring back good memories of childhood.

It is useful to know we have the capacity to self-soothe, and to recognise what our strategies are. In some situations, patients may feel so vulnerable and overwhelmed that they are unable to access their self-soothing strategies. Perhaps this is where complementary therapies involving repetitive soothing touch are helpful. In addition to offering a means of reducing the stress hormone cortisol, bodywork therapists are able to touch patients in a caring and nurturing way, and through their therapeutic skills are able to 'tune into the patient's need for calming'. As McFarland (1998, p.107) states, 'A kiss is just a kiss, a sigh is just a sigh, but the touch of a body worker...ahhh, that's something else.'

SELF-CARE

Although we may think of touch as physical contact with another person, there are many everyday situations where we are involved in self-touching. We need to wash/shower so we apply soap to our bodies, we groom ourselves, we wash our hair, we dress, and we feel the textures and the 'fit' of the clothes we are wearing. We choose clothes that feel right for an activity in terms of texture and style (not too tight or not too loose); we may apply creams, lotions and make-up (should we choose to do so). We need to know if our bedclothes are too warm or too heavy, which could stop us from sleeping. If we are shopping for personal items, we often need to 'touch' the fabric, or at least touch the surface of an item, before we consider making a purchase. Touch can also make a contribution to hobbies such as playing a musical instrument, embroidery, knitting, pottery, gardening, and many other pleasant pastimes. Some of these activities can contribute to self-soothing, although we may not realise it at the time.

A FEAR OF BEING TOUCHED

Receiving touch that is welcome is a basic human need at different stages of life. This kind of touch has a potency of its own. Unlike the other senses of sight, hearing, smell and taste that we can experience on our own, to experience 'interactive' human touch we need another person to be present. However, not all touch is welcome; the interpretation of the touch that is received may differ from the meaning that the giver had originally intended. Giving someone a hug may feel overwhelming for the recipient; putting an arm around someone's shoulders may be experienced as patronising, although the giver's intention was to be supportive. For some people, touch has no conscious meaning; there is acquiescence to receiving well-intentioned touch. The individual tolerates the touch merely to please another.

We do not like people who transgress the acceptability of certain social rules relating to touching. If we accidentally bump into someone in a shop or at a social event we immediately say, 'Sorry.' We are told 'Don't touch' in case we damage an object in a shop or we handle something without permission. Thumping, kicking, hitting, excessive tickling or using aggressive physical touch in bullying is unwanted and hurtful, and can make people fearful of touch. Possibly the worst form of touch, which can have devastating effects on an individual, is where touch is deliberately delivered in the form of physical and/or sexual violence. Just as good memories of receiving touch can be stored in the body, memories of unwanted, abusive touch can also be stored. There may be feelings of anger, frustration, fear and possibly sadness that need to be released. Often, people do not 'tell' of abuse, although it can contribute to poor physical health and low mental and emotional self-esteem. Abuse can also contribute to the use of unhelpful coping strategies, such as eating disorders, smoking, excess drinking of alcohol, self-harm or poor self-care (Bellis *et al*. 2014; Spratt *et al*. 2009). When emotions are associated with 'unwanted interference' and are not released, they can be directed inwards and stored in the body, possibly for many years (Upledger 1997).

However, in spite of physical abuse and the potential fear of receiving touch, there remains an innate need for humans to receive kind, well-intentioned touch. Smith, Clance and Imes (1998) suggest that although an abusive experience involving touch seems to produce a fear of being touched, a hunger for positive 'safe' touch remains. It may take time for such individuals to learn how to receive kind touch, to learn how to trust, and to maintain the trust with the person who is offering it. At the heart of reparative touch therapy there is a need for an individual to be in control of receiving the touch work. S/he needs to experience autonomy as a recipient, maintaining appropriate boundaries and consent throughout a touch experience.

Sadly, previous physical contact may not have been desirable and could be associated with harm and abuse, and such experiences may not be shared with a therapist or healthcare professional. There are some therapies involving touch that are designed to create and support emotional release, for example, biodynamic psychotherapy and craniosacral therapy. Sometimes patients may become tearful or be very guarded about where we can touch them. If a patient cries or becomes tearful during a treatment, it does not mean that that the release is due to a memory of trauma – it could be due to the sheer frustration or sadness with the current situation. However, we need to remember that the receiver of a touch therapy may have a history where connecting with positive touch can reawaken past nurturing experiences, and these memories can facilitate resilience in stressful situations.

PROFESSIONAL TOUCH

In clinical situations, Cocksedge *et al.* (2013) have defined 'procedural touch' as touch that is involved in a clinical task. They define 'expressive touch' as touch that is given freely and that is unrelated to a procedure/examination. Examples of expressive touch may involve holding a patient's hand, placing a hand on a patient's shoulder or giving a patient a hug. Ideally, expressive touch needs to take place where the giver is confident that it will be accepted.

Professionally, touch may be involved in a myriad of clinical procedures that healthcare professionals use in the course of their work. Throughout the cancer journey and depending on their roles, healthcare professionals are involved in touching patients. Doctors need to touch patients in the course of examinations, in administering some medical treatments and during surgery. Nurses may give injections, insert cannulas, arrange for intravenous treatments and change dressings. On the other hand, nursing assistants may be involved in washing patients and the more intimate sides of patient care... And then there are the physiotherapists, occupational therapists, radiographers and surgeons, all of whom will touch their patients in the course of consultations, examinations and treatments. There is much opportunity to offer kind, well-intentioned touch during the course of a patient's treatment and care.

TOUCH AS SENSORY LANGUAGE
AND METAPHOR

We often think that for touch to happen it needs to be a physical experience. However, the sense of touch is often incorporated into everyday verbal and written discourse, both as 'sensory language' and metaphor. The senses are often used in everyday language to describe a scene or an event. We absorb information about our experiences through our senses – visual, auditory, kinaesthetic (which involves touch, textures, feelings and movement), olfactory and gustatory. Examples of sensory words that describe touch and textures are soft, rough, smooth, hot, velvety, warm and cool. Sensory language can also be used therapeutically (see Chapter 5).

Metaphors are used to create an impact on the receiver; they aim to convey something more forcefully than an ordinary statement, and are an integral part of everyday sensory language. Knight (2002, p.125) has defined metaphors as 'symbols for what our unconscious mind is saying'. Sometimes they represent what we really want to communicate, and metaphors involving sensory language (see Chapter 5) help us to explain what we mean. Although we don't interpret the following phrases literally, it is likely we can interpret the meaning without difficulty. Some examples of metaphors relating to touch and kinaesthetic language are as follows:

I was very touched by his story.

He was very touchy this morning.

Stay in touch with me.

My manager is a bit of a soft touch.

I wouldn't touch it with a barge pole.

The pressure at the meeting was unbearable.

We gave her a warm welcome.

That feels like a good move.

This chapter began with a story about 'Ethel'. We will never know her touch history – or how many times she needed a hug, a cuddle or just someone to hold her hand. It does sound as though the quality of the touch she received from the carers in the centre was something new and different. The tragedy is that she felt she had to wait 80 years for the experience.

SUMMARY

This chapter has highlighted some aspects of touch that are not about techniques used in complementary therapies, but that are concerned with how we experience the powerful sense of touch in everyday life. The principles discussed have highlighted some of the areas that are pertinent to the work of complementary therapists and form a foundation for the remainder of the book.

Chapter 3

TOUCHING: AN EXPLORATION OF THE SKIN AND THE HANDS

KEYWORDS
touch; skin; hands; sensory cells; massage;
technology; HEARTS; Homunculus

INTRODUCTION

This chapter focuses on the structure and sensitivity of the skin and the human hand. The skin is the largest organ we have, and it is so highly innervated that it could be perceived as 'a sensory canvas'. As the complex properties and functions of the skin often go unrecognised, one of the main purposes of this chapter is to explore the structure of the skin and its sensitivity. Chemotherapy and other cancer treatments can affect the integrity and resilience of the skin; these conditions can present challenges for a massage therapist, with HEARTS offering a different approach. The use of a lubricant in massage and the role of fabric as an interface in HEARTS are explored. The unique structure, sensitivity and dexterity of the human hand are considered, together with the concept of Homunculus and the relationship between the brain and the hands. An exercise is included to help therapists develop their understanding of the principles of this relationship.

AN EXPLORATION OF THE SKIN

The skin has three layers – the epidermis, dermis and subcutaneous fat layer. The thickness of the epidermis (or outer layer) varies in different skin types. On the eyelids, the thickness is only 0.5 mm while on the palms and the soles of the feet the thickness is 1.5 mm. The dermis that is situated between the epidermis and the subcutaneous fat layer makes up 90 per cent of the skin and varies between a thickness of 1.5 mm and 4 mm. The subcutaneous fat layer is made up of adipose tissue, lymph vessels, hair follicles and blood vessels (Seer Training Modules, see National Cancer Institute 2018).

The skin is a remarkable organ; it covers the entire body, protecting it from infection, chemical agents and dehydration. Skin can self-repair and regenerate and has a role to play in the regulation of temperature through perspiration and shivering. Through a network of sensory cells the body is able to respond to different levels of pressure, pain, textures and temperature. The skin enables examination of some internal symptoms of the body through different degrees of palpation. Many therapies are carried out through the skin, such as osteopathy, polarity therapy, craniosacral therapy, shiatsu, Thai massage and biodynamic psychotherapy (see Further Reading and Online Resources).

In the context of HEARTS, it may be appropriate to think of our hands as a variety of 'paint brushes', and to regard the skin as a living 'sensory canvas' on which the hands can 'paint their art'. Although the skin appears 'flat', in reality it has weight and a large surface area as it covers the whole of the body. But what are the details of its structure? Anthropologist, Ashley Montagu (1986, p.7), outlines the physical properties of skin, the largest organ in the body, in Box 3.1.

Box 3.1. Physical structure of the skin

The surface area of the skin is approximately 19 square feet in the average adult male in whom it weighs 8 pounds. It contains some 5 million sensory cells, and constitutes some 12 per cent of body weight. The surface area of the skin has an enormous number of sensory receptors receiving stimuli of heat, cold, touch, pressure and pain. A piece of skin about the size of a dollar contains more than 3 million cells, 100–340 sweat glands, 50 nerve endings and 3 feet of blood vessels. It is estimated that there are some 50 receptors per 100 square millimetres, a total of 640,000 sensory receptors. The number of sensory fibres from the skin entering the spinal cord by the posterior roots is well over half a million.

It is the sensory cells that are of particular interest to the touch therapist. There is a huge network of sensory receptors and nerve endings throughout the skin. These enable us to detect stimuli that give rise to sensations such as temperature, pressure, pain, textures, movement and more...it is the group of sensory cells called mechanoreceptors that can detect textures, pressures and vibrations. There are four types of cells in this group that are related to touch, and the functions of these are outlined below:

- Merkel cells are able to sense light touch and are found in the basal layer of the epidermis. They can respond to very light touch and are found in glabrous regions of the skin, especially in the fingertips.

- Meissner's corpuscles are found in the dermis; they can adapt rapidly to different stimuli and also respond to light touch and changes in vibrations.

- Pacinian corpuscles are larger nerve plexuses that respond to mechanical stimuli of pressure and tension. They respond only to sudden disturbances and are particularly responsive to vibrations. These sensory cells are located deeper in the dermis.

- Ruffini corpuscles respond to touch, pressure and vibration, with mechanoreceptors responsible for sensing stretching, sustained pressure and perception of heat. These cells are also found deeper in the dermis.

In addition, there are thermoreceptors that respond to heat and cold, pain receptors that can detect injury or damage to the skin and proprioceptors that can sense different parts of the body in relation to each other.

The skin is sensitive enough to detect a gentle breeze or a minute change in temperature, although no obvious physical contact has apparently taken place. Rantala (2017) reports that the smallest detection threshold of weight is on the face, about 5 mg (i.e. 5/1000 g), which equals the wing of a fly dropping from a height of 3 cm onto the skin.

Properties of the skin that relate to touch therapy interventions, particularly massage

Healthy skin is very elastic and resilient; it is not too oily or too dry. When young, our skin is usually taut and supple, because the skin has an abundance of collagen and elastin. Collagen gives skin its structure, and elastin allows the skin to stretch. As we age, we produce less collagen and elastin, which is why the skin loses its resilience and elasticity. Additionally, many other factors affect skin health; these include sun damage, diet, pollution, smoking, trauma, medication and illness.

Swedish massage is a common approach to body massage, and forms the basis of massage training in many countries. One of its key characteristics is that the interaction between therapist and patient is usually through skin to skin, that is, the hands of the therapist are in direct contact with the skin of the patient. There is no separating interface between the two, apart from a lubricant, which can be either oil or cream. The aim of the repetitive (and usually enjoyable) massage is to ease muscle tension and promote circulation. Typically the treatment can last from 45 minutes to over an hour, although in cancer care the time may be shorter depending on the patient's condition.

The choice of lubricant depends on the aim of the massage and the condition of the skin. When oil is placed on the skin during massage, it will gradually be absorbed. The oil needs to provide sufficient 'grip' for the therapist and also permit a 'gliding' of the hands. The initial stroke, which is known as effleurage, is a firm, stroking movement, usually carried out in the direction of the venous and lymphatic flow, that is, towards the heart. Massage can be given at a variety of depths depending on its aim.

In cancer care, massage needs to be adapted to the patient's condition. The aim of the treatment, the amount of oil used, its density, the pressure applied, the adaptability of strokes chosen and the time spent with the patient must all be taken into consideration (Carter and Mackereth 2006). It is likely that massage is the complementary therapy that is most likely to be practised in supportive and palliative care (Mackereth *et al.* 2016).

Key challenges of using oils and creams in cancer care

There are challenges related to the condition of the skin for the massage therapist working in a cancer setting. Some of the most common challenges are outlined below:

- Cancer treatments, such as chemotherapy and steroids, may cause skin changes. These include dryness or inflammation that affect the rate of oil absorption.

- Skin irritation may occur due to the side effects of chemotherapy or radiotherapy.

- There may be profuse perspiration, possibly due to changes in body physiology, resulting in the oil becoming mixed with moisture on the skin's surface.

- The person may have cachexia, which is often associated with advanced cancer. Cachexia is a condition that is related to excessive weight loss, where both muscle and adipose tissue become diminished, leading to skin which has become 'loose'. (Dehydration can sometimes contribute to the presence of cachexia or loose skin.)

Of themselves, these conditions should not exclude massage, particularly if adaptions can be made; it is likely that patients still have a need to be touched in a kind, well-intentioned way (see Chapter 2). However, the need for touch could be satisfied through the use of HEARTS. Due to the use of a fabric interface between the therapist's hands and the patient's skin, HEARTS requires the hands to be used in a different way to massage; this is a different approach to 'massage through clothes and covers'.

Working though fabric does not permit the same 'grip and glide' of the hands as when a lubricant is used. However, a treatment can be offered in any place and at any time without having to find a lubricant; the patient does not need to remove any clothing; only light touch is used; and the skin is not directly touched by the therapist (see Chapter 6).

EXPLORING THE HANDS

At first sight, the hands are seemingly of a simple structure that enables us to do many actions, often without thinking. To remind us of this apparent simplicity, a picture of the hands is shown in Figure 3.1.

The hands are the main tools of all touch therapy practice, with great versatility and complexity. Each hand is made up of 27 bones, and in addition to the four fingers there is an 'opposable thumb'. The 'opposable thumb' is so called because it has the ability to be brought into an opposite movement to the fingers. Without the thumb, it would be almost impossible to grip, hold, or pick up small objects. The skin on the back of the hand is soft, thin and pliable, so when the fingers are stretched the skin can relax to accommodate the stretch. Conversely, when the fingers and thumb are flexed to make a fist, the skin is stretched across the muscles of the hand.

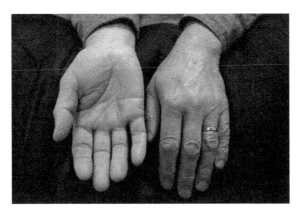

Figure 3.1. The hands are of an apparently simple structure, but this masks the incredible range of actions they are able to perform

The palm of the hand has in the region of 1700 touch receptors and free nerve endings that enable the hands to respond to pressure, movement and vibration. At the ends of the fingers are pads, from where fingerprints are obtained. This area is covered with papillary ridges that enable the ends of the fingers to act as surfaces which are involved in gripping, the sensitive holding of objects, applying very light pressure and sensing minute changes in textures. Skedung *et al.* (2013) suggest that human fingertips are probably the most sensitive skin areas in the animal world; the tips can feel the difference between a smooth surface and one with a pattern embedded just 10 nanometres deep. To give some meaning to the relationship of a nanometre to the sensitivity of the fingertips, a sheet of paper is around 100,000 nanometres in depth. (Interestingly, as technology advances, there is much work being carried out into the science of synthetic skin, computer touch screens and robotics. Investigations are ongoing into ways of replicating the sensitivity of the skin and the tiny movements of which the human hand is capable.)

However, the factor that probably gives the human hand its extra degree of sophistication is its direct connection to the neural anatomy of the brain and nervous system. Putz and Tuppek (1999, p.357) suggest that, 'the more recent evolution of the hand can be understood as the expression of the development of the brain. Therefore, the hand is a direct tool of our consciousness. It is a main source of differentiated tactile sensations as well as a precise working organ.' Goldschmidt and van Meines (2012, p.16) also refer to the sensitivity of the hands as being 'highly receptive in both giving and receiving touch'. They describe the hands as being the part of the body with which people feel most comfortable. There are many ways in which we use our hands, and while some suggestions are given in Box 3.2, this is by no means an exhaustive list.

Box 3.2. Activity range of the human hand

The human hand can make gestures that are expressions of our emotions and personalities. The range is vast, from demonstrating caring, affection, stroking, holding, tickling, hugging, kicking, hitting, scratching, punching...

- The handshake is a means of greeting, and possibly a means of saying goodbye. It is also a demonstration of closing an interaction, or where agreement has been reached, perhaps in the closing of a deal or course of action.

- Hands are a major sensory organ in distinguishing and experiencing textures. The receptors in the hands can detect sensations from sources that tell us about heat/ cold, wet/dry, rough/smooth, sharp/blunt, silky/hairy... All of these opposites can be placed on a continuum of extremes, and the receptors in the hands can detect and relay even the smallest of changes to the brain.

- Very intricate movements can be controlled and detected that make it possible for surgeons (and other healthcare professionals) to carry out the most intricate and delicate of procedures.

- The hands can play the most complex pieces of music on a variety of instruments. For example, a toccata is a piece of music which was originally written to demonstrate the speed, delicacy and intricacy of the movement of the fingers.

- Hands are capable of crafting, for example, embroidery, fine needlework, painting, calligraphy handwriting and pottery.

The properties of the hands as a sensory instrument are endless, and yet, as with other aspects of the sensory system, we tend to take them for granted. Gindrat *et al.* (2015) have reported that with the increase in touch screen use, there have been changes in the cortical areas of the brain, suggesting that our sensory areas are evolving with the repeated and skilled use of this technology. These changes are particularly noticeable where operating the technology requires the extensive use of the thumb, such as in texting.

The sensory receptors found on the palm of the hand and the fingertips are particularly effective in the Hands-on work of HEARTS. Most of the work is carried out with the palm of the hand with the thumb kept close to the hand so that the hand can be used as a single unit. If the thumb separates from the hand, the hand has a tendency to grip, which alters the tension in the hand when applying stroking movements. MacDonald (2014, p.102) also recommends a 'whole hands' approach for use in massage, and describes using the hands in this way as 'open, receptive and coaxing' (see Chapter 6).

THE HOMUNCULUS PRINCIPLE

In HEARTS, the sensory capacities of the hands are at the centre of the Hands-on work. If we were to express the size of the hands in relation to the rest of the body, they would seem relatively small and, in reality, they are not very large. However, if you take a look at Figure 3.2, you will notice that the size of the hands is very large in relation to other areas of the body. Other areas of the body also seem to be out of proportion. So how can this be?

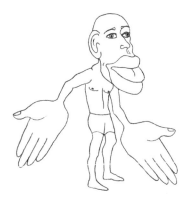

Figure 3.2. A visual representation of Homunculus (note the size of the hands in relation to the rest of the body)
Drawing by Fiona James

The data for this theoretical model was sourced during 126 brain operations, conducted under local anaesthetics by Dr Wilder Penfield between 1928 and 1936 (Penfield and Boldrey 1937). The results were collated and visually represented as a distorted human figure, known as the Homunculus (Catani 2017). The perceived large size of the hands is related to the density of sensory/motor receptors in the brain, not the anatomical area with which we are familiar. It is the density of these receptors which enables our hands to have their remarkable sensory properties. In the context of HEARTS, we would like readers to observe the relative size of the hands in relation to other parts of the body. It is interesting that when a therapist is working, s/he will often acknowledge that his/her hands feel larger during the treatment. Patients may share similar observations, referring to a part of their body that has received focused attention; for example, reporting an increase in the perceived size and awareness of the feet during reflexology.

Experimenting with the Homunculus principle

The aim of this exercise is to apply the theoretical principles to a 'HEARTS Homunculus Visualisation' (HHV). First, you, the therapist, need to observe the image of the Homunculus (see Figure 3.2) so you are familiar with the theoretical concept described above. It is probably easier to do if a friend reads the following instructions to you. Before you debrief, switch your roles so both of you have a turn at the visualisation.

1. First, I invite you to sit in a comfortable chair, with your eyes closed; then scan your own body in your mind's eye, from your feet to your head, becoming aware of the body's 'landmarks...' your feet...your lower legs...your knees... your thighs...your hips...your shoulders, and then your head...your arms...and your hands. (The landmarks form a sequence of places of the body and will be referred to throughout the book. They can be varied, depending on the situation.)

2. Now, place your hands on your thighs and gently apply light pressure as you breathe in, and then release the pressure as you breathe out. Repeat this process twice, and notice the size of your hands in your mind's eye and any warmth or coolness emanating from your palms. You may notice that

on the third practice of this process your hands feel bigger and there may be a temperature change in your palms. You are now engaging with your internal Homunculus.

3. Next, bring the hands upwards to shoulder height and turn the palms to face away from you. Breathe in with a comfortable breath as you stretch the fingers and then release the stretch as you breathe out. Repeat this process twice. Continuing with your eyes closed, become aware of the perceived weight, temperature and size of your hands. Now open your eyes to check out the image you hold in your mind's eye in relationship to what you observe as you look at the back of your hands.

4. Close your eyes again and bring your hands together, resting on your lap. Press them gently together as you breathe in, and then loosen the tension as you breathe out. Repeat this twice and then open your eyes and have a good stretch... you might experience a yawn(s) that is being triggered from engaging in this exercise. What do you notice about the size of your hands you experience in your mind? (This can also be a useful self-soothing exercise between patients.)

RECOMMENDATIONS

- When you do any Hands-on work maintain your awareness of how remarkable the skin and hands are. They are designed to work in harmony as skilled 'paint brushes' on a perfect 'sensory canvas'.

- When the skin and soft tissue are affected by illness or trauma, there is a need to use light, 'contactful' touch (which does not tickle), or even gentle holding or breeze strokes (see Chapter 6). The touch receptors in your hands will enable you to vary the sensitivity of the pressure and the speed you choose.

- If you wish, you can integrate HEARTS' other bodywork or massage sessions by working lightly over a blanket or towel with the hands. This approach could be used to begin or end a complementary therapy session, or it could be used as an interlude in the middle of a treatment.

SUMMARY

This chapter has reviewed the structure of the skin and hands as the key players in the physiological aspects of touching. The quality of the skin has been explored and the need for adapting massage has been discussed. This was followed by a brief description of some differences between massage and HEARTS. The Homunculus model has been used to explain the relationship between the brain and the hands. Whenever we work with touch, it is helpful to go 'beyond the technique' and remember that we are working with the 'whole person' through a remarkable sensory system.

Part 2

THE COMPONENTS
OF HEARTS

Chapter 4

EMPATHY

KEYWORDS
therapeutic relationships; empathy; compassion; sympathy;
intuition; empathic skills; compassion fatigue

INTRODUCTION

When the mnemonic HEARTS was devised, empathy was identified as a key element that served as a 'foundation' for all the other components. This chapter defines the 'therapeutic relationship' and describes some of the components of a successful therapeutic relationship. The potential contribution that empathy, compassion and sympathy can make to a therapeutic relationship is discussed. It is important that a therapist understands the difference between these three concepts, and is able to recognise how s/he is engaging with the patient (or carer). Reasons are given why therapists do not become involved in an empathic relationship with a patient, and suggestions made for developing empathic skills and ways of clearing thoughts and feelings about difficult situations.

DEFINING THE THERAPEUTIC RELATIONSHIP

First, it is important to define the term 'therapeutic relationship'. Cawthorn (2006, p.73) likens the relationship to a dance that is initiated and nurtured by the therapist. She suggests that some patients may immediately be 'in step', whereas others will actively 'take a step back' or 'sit this one out'. Cawthorn and Shepherd (2010, p.66) suggest that, 'A therapeutic relationship has, in its very existence, a commitment to the well-being of one person, the patient.' It is the role of the therapist to find resourceful ways of engaging with the patient, working towards a shared outcome. Orlinsky, Grawe and Parks (1994) identified several components that consistently have a helpful effect on treatment outcomes. These include the therapist's credibility and skill level, his/her empathic understanding, engaging the patient with regard to feelings and mood, and an affirmation of the patient's situation and concerns.

A touch-focused therapist may be involved with a patient for a short time. The first meeting may be the first and only time that s/he meets with that individual, particularly in a hospital setting. A high level of skill and confidence is needed to establish a relationship quickly, and to gain the patient's trust. Adding HEARTS to a therapist's skill set provides a therapeutic tool that can be helpful in a range of situations, and delivered in a short time frame. HEARTS provides an opportunity to be present for another, mindful of purpose, but not tied to clinical outcomes. For example, HEARTS cannot claim to eradicate pain, but could assist with increasing the patient's comfort and helping the patient to feel 'at ease'; the focus of the relationship is more akin to that of a helpful facilitator.

UNDERSTANDING EMPATHY, COMPASSION AND SYMPATHY

Empathy

Rothschild (2004) defined 'empathy' as the 'connective tissue' of good therapeutic practice. She argues that empathy is the factor that enables us to establish bonds of trust with patients, and to meet them with our hearts as well as our minds. In being empathic, the therapist seeks to understand a patient's distress from the individual's experience.

The word 'empathy' was derived from the German *einfühlung*, which is literally translated as 'feeling into' (Online Etymology Dictionary 2018). The therapist is able to put aside his/her own feelings, and demonstrate that s/he is able to be 'in the patient's shoes'. As a consequence, the patient feels valued, and that his/her problems are acknowledged and appreciated by the therapist on both cognitive and emotional levels.

Interestingly, Gallese *et al.* (1996) discovered that our brains are 'hardwired' to practise empathy. The researchers were studying grasping behaviour in monkeys; the monkeys' brain patterns were being monitored so that the researchers could identify which areas of the brain were activated when a monkey grabbed a raisin with its hand. During a rest period, one of the researchers reached for a raisin. To the surprise of everyone present, exactly the same neurons fired in the monkey's brain; it was as though the monkey was grasping a raisin at the same time!

The researchers discovered that a group of neurons (now called mirror neurons) actively fired when the monkey recognised what the researcher was doing. Further work enabled Gallese (2003) to hypothesise that sensations and emotions displayed by others can be empathised through a 'mirror-matching' mechanism in the brain. Gallese believed that we are born to resonate with each other, even at the deepest levels of emotion; as social and familial beings, we are able to connect and resonate with others. These physical and emotional responses, sometimes called 'body talk' or 'somatic resonance', can include yawning, laughing and crying in response to a shared experience (Bertolucci 2011; Ross 2000). On both a national and international level people can be moved to experience greater empathy for others at times of great loss or disasters, for example 9/11, school shootings or the death of a famous person. Perhaps this phenomenon explains the comments made by carers in Chapters 11 and 12 where the 'bystander effect' was experienced. When carers observed the therapists delivering HEARTS, they, too, experienced feelings of relaxation and calm, although they were not directly receiving any form of treatment.

Compassion

The word 'compassion' originates from the Latin *compassio*, which means 'to suffer with' (Online Etymology Dictionary 2018). Engel (2008) describes compassion as a desire to ameliorate, or at least reduce, the suffering of another person. Lilius *et al.* (2008) suggest that compassion could be perceived as a motivator to actively assist another in distress or difficulty, and Rogers (1951) suggests that compassion is motivated by unconditional positive regard for an individual. The terms 'empathy' and 'compassion' are often used interchangeably in healthcare, and there is some overlap and interaction between the between two. Sinclair *et al.* (2017) suggest that compassion enhances the key facets of empathy. Importantly, the additional component within compassion is the need to take action and do something to help. Compassion may be expressed with small acts of kindness that are 'extra' to the therapist's role.

Sympathy

Sympathy originates from the 1570s' French word *sympathie* and was originally translated as 'an affinity between certain things' (Online Etymology Dictionary 2018). Burton (2015) describes sympathy as 'a feeling of care and concern for someone' and Monroe (2002) states that sympathy is important in human relationships as an expression of concern or sorrow relating to a distressing event such as being made redundant, being diagnosed with a life-threatening illness or experiencing a bereavement. Clark (2010) suggests that to be sympathetic, it is not necessary to 'enter into' a patient's experience...it is possible to have only a general understanding of a patient's situation.

Unlike empathy, sympathy does not involve a shared perspective or shared emotions. The body language and tone of voice may imply caring and concern, but the therapist does not become involved further with the patient. If a therapist undertakes to form a therapeutic relationship from sympathy alone, the relationship is likely to be unproductive as the therapist will not have an understanding of the patient's needs, his/her feelings or emotions.

HOW DO PATIENTS RESPOND TO BEING RECEIVERS OF EMPATHY, COMPASSION AND SYMPATHY?

Do patients have an understanding of empathy, compassion and sympathy, and as receivers, can they tell the difference between the three? A study by Sinclair *et al.* (2017) involved 53 patients who were selected for having a terminal diagnosis and a life expectancy of less than six months. Semi-structured, individual interviews were conducted by an experienced research nurse in a private space within the hospital. The results are outlined in Box 4.1.

Box 4.1. Patients' responses to being receivers of empathy, compassion and sympathy

The patients had no difficulty in identifying the characteristics of empathy, compassion and sympathy, and were also able to voice how they felt when being on the receiving end of each of the three.

The patients recognised that empathy was much more than sympathy. They were able to sense that the interaction was empathic as they could 'feel it'. When a therapist entered an interaction from an empathic state, the patients felt acknowledged and supported. Empathy allowed for a deeper understanding of a patient's individualised suffering, and as a result, the patients felt confident that the therapist understood their individual situation and was personally involved.

The patients felt that compassion added something to the key components of empathy, and that empathy and compassion were beneficial. They also mentioned that where compassion was concerned, the healthcare provider would 'go above and beyond' and add to the care in ways that were not necessarily duty-based or remunerated.

While patients praised interactions of an empathic or compassionate nature, they were less complementary when they felt that someone was expressing sympathy. They said that they were left feeling demoralised, depressed and sorry for themselves, and disliked the 'pity-based' approach. They regarded sympathy as more about alleviating the distress of the observer rather than the distress of the patient.

RELUCTANCE TO ENTER INTO AN EMPATHIC RELATIONSHIP

In some situations, a therapist may feel that s/he would prefer to limit his/her involvement with the patient. The therapist may feel that s/he does not want to engage fully with an individual in case the interaction becomes overwhelming. Connecting with a patient may be reduced to protect the therapist from a feared abreaction or emotional outpouring. The therapist's responses may originate from over-involvement during previous clinical or complementary therapy practice. One way of avoiding too much involvement is for a therapist to talk about similar situations to those of the patient from his/her own experience, or to offer advice. Jeffrey (2016) has suggested that in order to relieve one's own distress, offering sympathy may take on a 'self-orientated' perspective. Sometimes the therapist may feel that s/he does not have the capacity to attend to, or assist with, the patient's difficulties. Other reasons may be linked to being time-poor, feeling inadequately prepared or feelings of a lack of support in the workplace (Booth *et al.* 1996).

Pressure to sustain empathic responses to patient suffering, without boundaries and support, may contribute to a risk of developing compassion fatigue and burnout. Compassion fatigue may be treatable, but being 'burnt out' may necessitate a change of role, a career break or even a career change in order to recover (Sabin-Farell and Turpin 2003). For the therapist to remain resilient, it is essential that s/he has strategies for avoiding a retention of emotions relating to empathic and compassionate relationships. Some suggestions for maintaining boundaries and releasing unresourceful thoughts are given later in this chapter.

THE ROLE OF EMPATHY IN HEARTS

HEARTS is an intervention that has empathy at its centre. Working with HEARTS has the potential to make the session a potent and memorable event – a resource in the moment and possibly for the future (see Chapter 12). An empathic relationship with a patient generates trust and bonding. Although empathy is a term usually applied to verbal interactions, it is essential that in HEARTS the principles of empathy (and compassion) also apply to the way in which the hands and the voice are used. Carter (2006, p.129) suggests that, 'empathy facilitates the use of intuition and creativity on the part of therapist and patient, so that each component can be applied in harmony with another, thus producing a synergistic effect. In HEARTS, touch and empathy are fundamental and intertwined, one cannot be offered without the other.'

The ability to choose and apply each component in harmony with another helps to facilitate a synergistic effect for the patient (and bystanders). Therapists need to be aware of the emotional power of the hands to convey non-verbal messages that may include caring, support, safety and a 'compassionate willingness' to do something that could help. I encourage all therapists to remember that hands can communicate 'very eloquently' when we are truly present with another person. For patients who are not used to receiving kind, respectful and thoughtful touch (or who have a 'hunger for it'), the initial contact alone may be enough to create an emotional response. HEARTS can offer a shared 'whole person' experience, which, in turn, can create new 'sensory memories' as a resource for now and for the future.

So how can this be achieved? When a therapist feels confident in using the skills involved in HEARTS, s/he will be able to use intuition to tailor the work to a patient's physical and emotional needs. Sometimes, when intuition is discussed, a therapist may think that s/he can touch anywhere on the patient's body as it is 'intuitive'. This is not good practice – using your intuition must be based on sound therapeutic principles and duty of care. Offering choice acknowledges that an individual's permission and preferences are important and to be respected. Additionally, we need to work within the boundaries of the contract we agree with the patient.

DEVELOPING EMPATHIC SKILLS

Studies involving nurses have demonstrated that empathy can be developed and enhanced. Cunico *et al.* (2012) conducted a study of student nurses studying on a three-year degree course. Data was collected using the Italian version of the Balanced Emotional Empathy Scale (BEES). Students in the Intervention Group attended additional seminars and workshops to develop communication and empathic abilities. Data showed that the training was especially effective for women. At the end of three years the scores increased from a baseline of 31.60 to 42.91.

Therapists' skills sets vary and there is always need for review and development. So how can therapists enhance their empathic skills? The following suggests some ways of developing empathy within a therapeutic relationship.

1. Know your values

First, have you recognised your values when working in a supportive care setting? Values represent what is important to you, for example, kindness, humour, compassion, truth, wisdom, honesty. Your values are qualities that are not physical, you cannot touch them, but you will have them with you all the time. An exercise that you may want to do with a friend is as follows: write down ten values that underpin your practice as a therapist, and then share your list with a friend who has also written down ten values. Don't interrupt each other until you have reached the end of your lists.

2. Establish rapport

Rothschild (2004) suggests that empathy is felt in the body and not in the mind. Perhaps the first step is to understand the importance of body language in establishing rapport with the patient. Rapport is a process that is established when the therapist uses his/her body language, tone of voice and the words s/he uses to mirror those of the patient's. This is a powerful process that enables the therapist to put him/herself in someone else's shoes.

There are many aspects of body language that a therapist can mirror without it being overt mimicking. We need to bear in mind that when we are getting on with someone and having a really interesting conversation, it is very likely that we would be mirroring each other without even thinking about it.

Some body positions that are easy to mirror are:

- Face, for example facial expressions

- Posture, for example upright, relaxed

- Angle of the head, for example tilted, bending forward, staring at the ceiling

- Arms, for example folded, loosely by the side

- Hands, for example relaxed or tense, shoulders hunched, hand gestures

- Legs, for example crossed or apart

- Feet, for example relaxed, toes pointed, constant tapping or feet moving up and down.

It is also helpful to match the tone and level of the voice. Once the body language is matched it will be much easier to match the tone and volume of the patient's voice. While our body language may be mirroring the other person's, there may be a difference in other aspects of our interaction, for example, frequently looking at the clock or being distracted by outside noises. This is known as incongruence, and it is important to remember that just as we are attempting to mirror the patient's body language, s/he will also be receiving and interpreting the non-verbal signals we are sending. If there is incongruency, this is likely to be detected by the patient. Similarly, if a therapist is suggesting reflexology and the person is saying 'Yes, that would be nice' but something tells the therapist that the patient is demonstrating incongruency, other options may need to be offered.

3. Recognise rapport in everyday life

Establishing rapport is a useful skill to develop. Observing the rapport you may have with a friend will help you to recognise what is happening between yourself and a patient. Next time you are in a social situation, perhaps having a chat over coffee, notice when you are in rapport with your friend. You may find that as you lean back in your chair, your friend does the same, or you both find yourselves nodding or stirring your coffees at the same time. This can be a fun exercise – sometimes your friend will follow your 'lead' and sometimes you will follow your friend's movements.

4. The role of an observer

You could shadow a trusted colleague to discover how s/he establishes empathy with patients. (It would be helpful if you could do this with a HEARTS therapist, if possible.) Alternatively, you may like to ask a trusted colleague to give you some constructive feedback on one of your sessions. If you choose to do this in a clinical setting, you will need to gain the patient's permission to have a third person present.

5. The value of reading

In the References list at the end of this book and the Further Reading and Online Resources there are some very good articles on the topics described in this chapter. Do investigate, as the content is relevant to the main points raised in this chapter.

STAYING RESILIENT AND RESOURCEFUL

Carter and Mackereth (2017) have identified that the ability to remain resilient and resourceful is an essential attribute for therapists. Being 'resilient' may be defined as 'the ability to withstand or recover from difficult conditions'. Resourcefulness could be described as 'having the ability to spring back and to overcome difficulties' (*Concise Oxford English Dictionary* 2006).

Working with patients and carers can be very rewarding, but we may begin to take some of our patients' stories and their distress home with us. If this pattern of gathering a patient's problems persists, it can overwhelm us. Eventually we may realise we have fallen into a state of mind called the 'compassion trap'. It may happen that if we weren't comfortable with an outcome, we may 'try even harder' next time. Developing a thought pattern of 'not being good enough' is not resourceful. To avoid this state of mind building, it is important to clear our thoughts between one patient and the next, and to be compassionate towards ourselves.

Some suggestions for staying resilient and resourceful are outlined below:

- It is all too easy for kind, compassionate therapists to want to support a patient, but then we may begin to 'take the patient's problems home' with us. The mind has a very vivid imagination, and we can find ourselves inventing solutions, scenarios and outcomes for our patients. The only person who can resolve the patient's problems is the patient. We can help them to become resourceful and resilient, but we cannot 'fix' it for them. So leave stories and events that don't belong to you at work – both you and your patients have your own individual paths to follow.

- The past is gone and you cannot rewind time to start again. Remember that it takes two people to make a successful treatment, and a patient has the choice as to the extent to which s/he engages with the treatment and the therapist.

- Use your hand washing routine to wash away any unhelpful thoughts about the previous treatment, your relationship with the patient and the outcome of the treatment.

- If you are working in one room, clear the space and remake the bed before the next person enters so that the space is refreshed, and begin again.

- Arrange some clinical supervision, which can range from 45–60 minutes on a monthly basis, or a shorter time of perhaps 15 minutes, to address a specific issue.

- Use the Butterfly Hug described in Box 4.2 that simulates the wings of a butterfly. This method is used extensively for helping to process trauma and crises and during the standard protocol for the Eye Movement Desensitisation Realisation (EMDR) process. The principles can be used in a variety of situations where there is a need to self-calm or self-soothe.

This approach can be helpful to reduce unhelpful thoughts, feelings and associations. Luber (2009) suggests that when any negativity has been reduced, it is easier to develop more realistic formulations about a patient's future therapy. Positive, creative thinking can proceed without feelings of unease, weariness and ineffectiveness being present in the background. It is important to deal with any residual or negative feelings as they arise. Such feelings must not be allowed to accumulate as they can have detrimental effects on health and cause career burnout.

Box 4.2. The Butterfly Hug

If you are unfamiliar with the Butterfly Hug, adopt the arm and hand positions as shown in the image below.

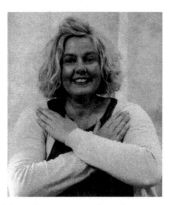

Arm and hand positions for the Butterfly Hug

Without moving the hand positions, slowly and gently tap each side alternately. Continue this alternating sequence until you are at ease with maintaining 10–15 taps on each side of the body. Once you have established a steady rhythm, you are ready to begin the process.

1. First, bring up the image of the patient in your mind's eye. (If you notice the image fades, which can happen, just bring it back again when you become aware of its absence.)

2. Do 10–15 Butterfly Hugs.

3. Notice whatever positive thoughts come to mind. Typically, this is something like 'I'm doing the best I can' or 'I can handle this' or 'It's good enough.'

4. Now install the positive thoughts with the patient's image. You can say the positive words aloud or in your head while you hold the image.

5. Do 10–15 Butterfly Hugs.

6. What do you notice?

Repeat the process, if necessary.

SUMMARY

The therapeutic relationship has been defined and the principles that underpin the concepts of empathy, compassion and sympathy have been discussed. The presence of empathy as a key component of the therapeutic relationship and any touch and voice work that is offered to a patient has been recommended. It is likely that patients will have an understanding of empathy, compassion and sympathy in the delivery of healthcare. Some suggestions for recognising and developing empathy skills have been suggested. It is important for therapists to be resourceful and resilient, and some resources for achieving these have been included. Finally, remember to be compassionate towards yourself and towards your work.

Chapter 5

RELAXATION

KEYWORDS
relaxation; stress; response; distress; eustress; person-centred
guided imagery (PCGI); sensory language; noisy environments

INTRODUCTION

The purpose of this chapter is to provide a foundation for the principles of the relaxation process (details of the applications in the HEARTS Process are given in Chapters 7 and 8). First, different interpretations of the process of relaxation are discussed and reference is made to the stress response and the roles of the sympathetic and parasympathetic nervous systems. The principles of good practice in delivering a resourceful relaxation session are explained. These include the use of sensory language and an invitational approach. Examples of some unresourceful phrases are included, together with more resourceful alternatives. Person-centred guided imagery (PCGI) is explained (and advocated), and examples of research relating to guided imagery are given in table form. A key challenge for therapists is working in busy and noisy environments, and strategies are suggested for accommodating or overcoming this, with recommendations given at the end of the chapter.

THE AIM OF RELAXATION WITHIN THE HEARTS PROCESS

The aim of HEARTS is to help a patient to achieve a state of calm, reduce 'distress' and contribute to a patient's resilience. The processes involved in HEARTS encourage the purposeful stimulation of the parasympathetic (calming) nervous system through the skilful use of touch and, when appropriate, the use of person-centred guided imagery (PCGI) and/or music. If we ask a patient what s/he does to counteract stress, they are unlikely to say that they use a complementary therapy. Some responses to this question are detailed below.

PATIENTS' DIFFERENT INTERPRETATIONS OF RELAXATION

When we ask a patient what s/he does to relax, the answer(s) will probably be about everyday activities, for example, 'I have a coffee with a friend', 'I watch TV', 'I phone someone for a chat', 'I go in the garden', 'I walk the dog' – or 'I have a drink.' When asked about the benefit(s) of the activity, the patient will probably respond with 'It takes my mind off worrying', 'I enjoy it', 'It makes me feel better' or 'I feel normal again.'

A metaphor is often used in place of the word 'relax'; we frequently hear people refer to doing something they enjoy as 'to chill'. 'To chill' could imply that the 'heat' needs to be taken out of a situation; this can be achieved by refocusing on something that is contrasting and engaging, which brings pleasure and involvement. Whichever method of 'chilling' is chosen, it is likely that there will be a calming effect on the physiology of the body, or on the chatter of the mind, at least in the short term. When patients are coping with multiple stressors it is all too easy for them to forget about the small things that they enjoyed when they were well. It can be helpful for patients to be reminded of these activities, and if they are no longer able to be involved physically in an activity, they may be encouraged to seek something new, as a way of self-soothing and managing stressors.

However, when patients are about to receive a procedure, such as a cannulation or injection, most are at least apprehensive, or so fearful that they panic. Unhelpful phrases such as, 'You will feel a short, sharp scratch; just relax for me please' or 'It will be much easier if you relax and stay calm' do nothing to calm the patient. Simple breathing techniques may be offered at the time of an intervention, which may have a calming effect. If the patient has learned a relaxation technique such as progressive muscle relaxation, guided imagery or mindfulness, s/he could be encouraged to use this during the intervention.

Relaxation can be many things to many people. Not knowing what is meant by relaxation – or how to achieve it – can become yet another stressor! In the context of HEARTS, relaxation may be defined as 'a conscious physical and mental state, which encompasses a process of becoming calm, lowering anxiety and reducing tension, which may be accompanied by a temporary period of peace and tranquillity'. The state of relaxation is not permanent, but it can help to prepare a person for a challenging episode or to create a break in a period of ongoing stress, for example, caring for someone who is seriously ill. Experiencing relaxation can literally 'recharge the batteries', and be a resource that can be recalled to help with self-soothing, so promoting resilience.

PHYSIOLOGICAL RESPONSE TO STRESSORS

The body's ability to respond to stressors is a natural part of our survival mechanism. In prehistoric times, the purpose of the 'stress response' was to respond to an event that could be life-threatening. This response has persisted throughout history. When a threat was perceived, rapid physiological changes were triggered in the body that enabled an individual to either fight the threat or flee. This is a very useful response to have when the threat is real – it could be a life saver. The downside is that in the 21st century, the mind doesn't always distinguish between a real threat and an imagined threat – the fight/flight response remains the same. Patients are usually relieved to learn that, in this respect, they are just like everyone else, and the stress response is common to everyone.

Although many of the stressors involved in cancer care aren't immediately life-threatening, they can generate unpleasant reactions, both physically and mentally. The stressors are not only concerned with treatments and medical procedures; they can be associated with family, friends, relationships, jobs, money concerns...the list is specific to an individual, as no two people respond to a situation in exactly the same way. The fight/flight response is described in a story form in Box 5.1. This story has been used to explain to patients about how we are 'hardwired' for a strong, and often unhelpful, stress response.

Box 5.1. The story of the stress response

A warrior sits on a rock as the sun goes down (no computer, no television, no mobile phone). Suddenly, there is a rustle in the bushes and immediately the stress response kicks in and the sympathetic nervous system is activated. First, adrenaline is released and this triggers the body's chemical reactions to either fight or flee the sabre-toothed tiger. Hearing becomes more acute and the pupils widen to let in more light. Muscles tense in readiness, and the demand for nutrients and oxygen increases as 'fuel' for the muscles. Nutrients and energy in the form of sugars are released from glycogen in the liver. The breathing rate increases, bringing more oxygen into the body; the heart rate speeds up to send the blood, containing the 'fuel', to the muscles, to prepare them for fight or flight. Additionally, the warrior may experience 'butterflies', which is due to the release of adrenaline and the creation of increased alertness. The skin sweats to cool the body, and there will be a need for the body to become 'lighter'.

In the 21st century the way the body can become lighter is to visit the toilet, but in prehistoric times, perhaps any place would do! Three other factors that may not be visible also occur – the blood-clotting factor increases to heal wounds and the immune system and digestive systems temporarily close down. Our warrior decides that the sabre-toothed tiger is too large to fight, so to survive he hides in a cave. Keeping very still, he sees the sabre-toothed tiger sauntering past. On this occasion the animal is not a danger at all, but the warrior has learned that a sabre-toothed tiger is a real and present danger – with a risk of being eaten alive – and so the body responds accordingly. As the immediate danger passes, his parasympathetic nervous system (which does the calming) is initiated, and the body's chemicals are restored to a state of balance. Our warrior feels elated to live another day.

Chemical effects of the stress response

Adrenaline is of two kinds – noradrenaline, which stimulates fight, anger and aggression, and adrenaline, which stimulates flight, fear and withdrawal. Alongside the production of adrenaline is a chemical called cortisol that causes depression and feelings of loss of control. If any of these substances can be reduced, the patient is likely to feel more comfortable and will be able to return to a more balanced state. Looker and Gregson (1991) suggest that where there is a sufficient decrease in noradrenaline/adrenaline and cortisol, the individual may enter a state of relaxation, calm and serenity.

Although the word 'stress' is most commonly used, it may be more accurate to identify the effects of some stressors as causes of 'distress'. There is another kind of stress that is less well known, called 'eustress'. Eustress is the 'good' state we experience when we have achieved something that was a challenge to us. It is an event, or experience, which took us outside our comfort zone. In the context of cancer, examples of eustress may be learning to cope with the fear of radiotherapy treatment, getting through a scan using calming techniques, and being given the 'all clear' by a consultant. Eustress leads to a state of elation that is caused by an increase in testosterone (in both males and females) and a lowering of cortisol.

Although the parasympathetic nervous system is auto-matically initiated to rebalance the chemicals that cause the (dis) stress response, we do not have to rely solely on the absence of stressors to trigger it. It is the calming nervous system that is of particular interest to touch therapists; therapies such as guided imagery, massage and reflexology are known to reduce adrenaline and cortisol (Charalambous *et al.* 2016; Field 2014; Tiran and Mackereth 2010). It may be useful for a patient to be aware that s/he can initiate the calming nervous system by self-soothing (see Chapter 2), or by using such techniques such as progressive muscle relaxation, mindfulness or meditation. Initially, if using a complementary therapy, patients will require a treatment from a therapist, but adapted techniques may be learned by a carer (see Chapter 10). Alternatively, the patient can recall the sensations and the 'feeling good' factor triggered by the treatment for use when the therapist is not available as a form of self-help.

RECOGNISING THE RELAXATION RESPONSE

Just as we can recognise symptoms of stress, such as agitation, tension, disturbed sleep, rapid heart rate, dry mouth and nausea, so we can learn to recognise when the calming nervous system has been activated and the relaxation response is taking place. Carter and Mackereth (2010) identified some of the principle physiological changes that may be observed when a patient enters a state of calm or a state of relaxation:

- Conversation ceases
- Full eye closure
- Rapid eye movements
- A deep sigh
- Breathing slows
- Increased salivation (dribbling)
- Increased peristalsis (tummy rumbles)
- Physical relaxation of muscles, involuntary movements such as twitching
- Tearing in the eyes
- Crying/laughing
- Flatus/burping.

During a therapy session, when we recognise that physiologically a patient is becoming more relaxed, it could be helpful to acknowledge the changes and to encourage the patient to become aware of them. A useful phrase that a therapist could use that can help promote an even deeper relaxation is '…and notice how your body is entering a more relaxed state, with tension melting… I am noticing your breathing appears to be more comfortable and your shoulders are more at ease…' It is amazing how the body knows how to make the most of relaxation.

WORKING WITH A PATIENT-CENTRED APPROACH

While acknowledging that there are many different methods of promoting relaxation, guided imagery has become a popular method of using the voice as it is easy to engage the 'chattering mind', which patients often talk about. The therapist's voice can be used as a 'sensory commentary' that accompanies the Hands-on work (see Chapter 7). Alternatively, some guided imagery using a patient's narrative relating to an aroma can be used (see Chapter 8).

Buckle (2003) suggests that the cancer journey can feel like a 'pathless path' – the patient is on a continual journey of hospital visits, diagnostic tests and treatments, with uncertainty about the outcome. Often, patients can feel that they have little choice in what is happening to them. Working in a patient-centred way can help the individual to feel that s/he has some control and a role to play in his/her treatment (Carter and Mackereth 2017). Some examples of how a patient could have some input into a HEARTS treatment are:

- Arranging the couch and the pillows.

- Choosing a texture with which to be covered, where possible (see Chapter 6).

- Giving feedback on the strokes using a hand signal, for example, the 'thumbs up' sign.

- Having the opportunity to tell the therapist if there is anything that s/he does not like or want, for example, having the head stroked, abdominal work or work on the feet.

- Devising his/her personal narrative (past, present or future) for relaxation.

- Giving feedback to the therapist at the end of the treatment (if awake).

- Giving permission for a carer to be present.

RESPONDING TO THE PATIENT'S PHRASE 'IT'S FINE'

When a therapist has done his/her best to make the patient comfortable, such as supporting the patient's knees or ankles with a pillow or rolled towel, s/he is likely to ask the patient, 'How is that for you?' The patient will probably respond with, 'It's fine', which may really mean, 'It's okay, but the pillow is too high, I don't really need it – and I would like you to take the towel away…but I don't want to disappoint you, or be a nuisance, so I will say it's okay.' Sometimes, open-ended questions (those that begin with how, who, what, where, when and why) are favoured as they have a reputation for promoting an 'open conversation'. In this situation, the therapist does not need an in-depth conversation; all s/he needs to know is if the action has increased the patient's comfort or otherwise. Although closed questions are thought to be more limiting as they can invite one- or two-word answers, in this situation, a closed question can be more useful in arriving at the optimum comfort level. For example, when the position of a pillow is changed, the patient can be asked, 'Is this better or worse?' If the patient says, 'It's worse', the therapist can then ask, 'What needs to happen to make it better for you?' and then the patient is able to give a more resourceful answer as to what s/he would really like.

HELPING TO CREATE A RESOURCEFUL RELAXATION EXPERIENCE

The following characteristics may contribute to a resourceful HEARTS session:

- The therapeutic relationship needs to be built on empathy and trust (see Chapter 4).

- The patient needs to understand the process and to give his/her consent.

- S/he needs to be comfortable, warm and covered with a suitable texture (chosen by the patient when possible).

- The therapist needs to understand and accept the patient's physical and emotional state.

- The length of time for which a patient can stay in one position needs to be assessed.

- The treatment needs a beginning, active treatment and a conclusion.

- The session should be kept short and effective – possibly between 5 and 20 minutes.

- The patient should be monitored by observing his/her physical responses, especially on the face. (Therapists should avoid focusing on their hands for the duration of the intervention!)

- The therapist should use invitational language, and where possible, the words of the patient (see Chapter 7).

- If the patient falls asleep, a nurse/carer needs to know that the patient has been left sleeping.

PERSON-CENTRED GUIDED IMAGERY SESSION

King (2010) suggests that patients should be allowed to create their own place or image of relaxation and peacefulness. Person-centred guided imagery (PCGI) means that the patient designs his/her imagery narrative; and the therapist provides a framework encouraging the patient to construct his/her personal scenario using sensory language. There is a growing body of evidence for using PCGI with a variety of clinical conditions (see Table 5.2).

The general language of promoting relaxation is really important – the process is one of offering invitations and suggestions to the patient, rather than giving a series of commands. There are some useful principles that demonstrate good practice in constructing relaxation sessions. The first is the use of a sensory language framework, and the second is the choice of words and phrases we use to encourage resilience and resourcefulness. (Three approaches to HEARTS that have patient involvement are described in Chapter 7, and a method for constructing PCGI using aromas and the patient's narrative is described in Chapter 8.)

Using a sensory framework

Images are formed in the brain through receiving nerve impulses from our physical senses. These are:

- Visual: the images shape the scenery and colours that we see

- Auditory: the sounds we hear

- Kinaesthetic: touch, textures, movement, emotions and sensory experiences

- Olfactory: aromas and the scents we smell

- Gustatory: the flavours we taste.

These five senses are often referred to by the mnemonic VAKOG, which is just a convenient 'word' for remembering what the five senses are. It is possibly more helpful for the therapist if s/he thinks of the five senses as a 'sensory framework' from which we can help the patient to construct his/her guided imagery narrative (see Chapter 8). Some examples of sensory language that we use in everyday speech are listed in Table 5.1. The lists refer to the first three senses of VAKOG, which are the ones we use most frequently.

Table 5.1. Some examples of sensory language

Visual	Auditory	Kinaesthetic
see	hear	feel
picture	tell	rough
bright	loud	smooth
colour	talk	touch
clear	bang	silky
focus	sound	fluffy
sparkle	pitch	cool
perspective	muffled	hot
view	ring	dance

The other two senses, olfactory and gustatory, are not as widely used in everyday language as the three described above, although they can be included in the patient's narrative if the situation requires.

Battino (2000) states that people have a preferred way of representing their experiences to the world through language. The three senses outlined above are the three significant 'representational systems'. It is possible that a person who has a kinaesthetic lead system and who likes to use words from the kinaesthetic column will find it more difficult to access visual images or to see pictures in their minds. If we include a patient's own imagery system, we are using the sensory language in a way with which the patient is familiar. For example, if a patient has a primary lead system that is visual, it is possible that s/he will find it easier to tell the therapist about what s/he sees rather than what s/he hears. One system is not better or more effective than any of the others; in practice it is likely that we will use words from all the representational systems.

Resourceful and invitational language

In helping people to drift into a relaxation state, the use of resourceful language is paramount, as some words or phrases may trigger unpleasant responses and memories. Using language that gives the patient choice(s) through invitation or suggestion is more acceptable than giving commands. Some examples of 'commands' together with examples of resourceful language are given below:

1. 'Take three deep breaths for me, please'

First, what is a 'deep breath'? If someone has breathing problems, a 'deep breath' can be very scary. We are asking the person to pay attention to his/her breathing to slow down the breathing rate 'for me'. Adding 'for me' implies that the patient is taking 'three deep breaths' for the benefit of the therapist, whereas the intention is that the 'deep breaths' are for the benefit of the patient.

Suggestion: 'You may like to notice each breath...and as you continue breathing in a rhythm which is comfortable for you...you may begin to notice that as you listen to my voice...your breathing may become a little slower...'

2. 'Get as comfortable as you possibly can'

This phrase implies that there is an ultimate goal – that of 'maximum' comfort. Adding 'as you possibly can' implies that the patient may not be able to achieve this goal and that there will be more to do in terms of achieving 'maximum comfort'.

Suggestion: '...and if you wish...you may like to adjust your position so that you feel even more comfortable...so that it becomes even easier for you to relax...'

3. 'Now, close your eyes'

Not everyone wants to close their eyes when they are told to do so. It may be scary to 'close down' your visual sense, and some people do not close their eyes until some time later in the session – if at all.

Suggestion: 'You may like to close your eyes...and, of course, you may keep them open if you wish...it is your choice to decide when you want to close your eyes...' A second option is to say, 'You may notice your eyelids becoming heavy...you may want to resist and watch what I am doing if you choose...and then when you are ready, let your eyes close...' If you want to add some playfulness, you could always add '...and you can peek...and see what is happening at any time'.

4. 'For the next two minutes, concentrate on focusing on your breathing'

If taken literally, 'two minutes' is a long time, and it is unlikely that the therapist really means 'two minutes'. 'Concentrate on focusing' implies a sustained effort and it is also difficult to interpret the meaning behind this phrase; it is also a direct instruction.

Suggestion: 'Can I invite you to notice your breathing...from time to time...so that you are breathing in a way that is comfortable for you?'

5. 'Perhaps you can see yourself on a lovely warm beach on a desert island'

This is far too specific – not everyone likes a beach, and the thought of being on a desert island would be horrific for some people. A desert island could suggest loneliness and being afraid that you might not be rescued. An open approach is more resourceful.

Suggestion: '...and you may like to let yourself drift to a place where you feel comfortable and at ease...a place which holds good memories...or somewhere where you would like to visit...'

WORKING IN NOISY ENVIRONMENTS

Have you noticed that in a noisy environment, such as at a party or a conference, when you become fully engaged with an individual with whom you have a shared interest, the noise is less noticeable as a 'connection' takes over?

On occasions, all therapists work in areas that may have an increased degree of noise and activity, especially if the therapist is working on a busy ward, a chemotherapy suite or a radiotherapy unit. In addition to working with a patient who may be distressed, there is background noise and interruptions. Treatment schedules may be changed, doctors may need to see the patient urgently, and sometimes it is difficult to understand how anyone can enter a state of relaxation at all. But it is possible! Position yourself where the patient can hear you, so instead of beginning at the feet, you may need to start at the patient's shoulders or arms. Acknowledge the noise by saying something like, 'You may be aware of the noise, it is coming from nurses helping patients, and visitors coming to see their loved ones... I would like to invite you to listen to my voice...

as we start the HEARTS session, I will be explaining to you how my hands are working...'

Details of a commentary that you can use where there is a noise 'overload' are given in Chapter 7.

RECOMMENDATIONS

- Explore the concepts of stress and the body's responses so you are confident to explain these principles quickly and easily to patients, for example, creating your own warrior story.

- Investigate sensory language and how we construct images – a useful book, NLP at Work, is detailed in Further Reading and Online Resources.

- Wherever possible, invite the patient to learn and practise some techniques for resourceful self-soothing as a result of your session with them.

- In noisy environments, commit to your intention and continue to engage with the patient. Once s/he is engaging with you and the work, the noise will become less intrusive and could be acknowledged within the narrative.

- Identify opportunities for working with PCGI within your developing practice.

- Practise using resourceful, invitational language with a friend/colleague; it is much easier and more fun to generate phrases if there are two of you.

SUMMARY

Promoting relaxation and a sense of calm is a pleasant and beneficial experience for therapists and patients. Different interpretations of relaxation have been described and concepts of distress and eustress have been discussed. A brief overview of the physiological processes involved to prepare the body for fight/flight have been included. Much of the chapter has focused on good practice and working in a patient-centred way. The use of sensory frameworks and working with the patient's narrative have been recommended.

Table 5.2. Guided imagery (GI) research

Study	Objective	Design	Outcome measures	Results	Comments on the intervention(s)
Patricolo *et al.* (2017)	To determine whether massage or GI could reduce pain and anxiety and improve sleep	Convenience sample with recruitment to two groups – the massage group (*n*=243) or GI (*n*=45)	Massage pre- and post-anxiety and pain scales. Survey with regard to pain, anxiety and insomnia for GI participants	Significant reduction in self-reported measures in both groups Poor recruitment to the GI group – authors suggested greater education needed for clinical staff	GI script focused on permission to relax, working with breath, taking control of fears and anxiety, washing away pain, a healing sun sending warmth to areas of discomfort or pain and accessing a beautiful, peaceful place to promote sleep, wonderful dreams and promoting ability to return to sleep, if disturbed
Shahriari *et al.* (2017)	To evaluate the effect of progressive muscle relaxation (PMR), GI and deep diaphragmatic breathing on the quality of life (QoL) in older people with cancer	Randomised controlled trial (RCT) (*n*=50) Combined interventions and usual care control groups	European Organisation for Research and Treatment of Cancer and QoL Questionnaire – core questionnaires completed before and six weeks after the intervention for the patients in both groups	There was statistically significant improvement in QoL and physical functioning post the combined interventions	Patients were asked to visualise the scenery that was the most pleasant to them for 10–15 minutes Researchers argued that the combining of GI with PMR and deep breathing was for its synergetic effects

cont.

Study	Objective	Design	Outcome measures	Results	Comments on the intervention(s)
Charalam- bous *et al.* (2016)	To test the effectiveness of GI and PMR on a cluster of symptoms experienced by patients receiving chemotherapy	RCT with participants (*n*=208) equally assigned, either in the intervention or the usual care control group	Patients were assessed for pain (0–10 scale), fatigue (CFS), nausea, vomiting and retching (INVR), anxiety (ZSRS) depression (DBI-11) and patients' self-reported health-related quality of life (HRQoL)	Patients in the intervention group experienced lower levels of *fatigue* and pain compared with those in the control group, and experienced better QoL	Patients experienced four weeks of weekly supervised and daily unsupervised sessions of GI and PMR based on a script with suggestions about auditory, tactile and olfactory images, and accompanied by soft music camouflaged with alpha waves pulses
Forward *et al.* (2015)	To investigate the effectiveness of the 'M' technique, method of structured touch using a set sequence and number of strokes, and a consistent level of pressure on feet and hands, compared with GI and usual care, in patients undergoing elective total knee or hip replacement surgery	Three-group RCT (*n*=225), with 75 in each	Reduction of pain and anxiety post-operatively Secondary outcomes measured use of pain medication and patient satisfaction	M showed the largest decreases in both pain and anxiety between groups No significant difference in narcotic pain medication use between groups Patient satisfaction survey ratings were highest for M, followed by GI	The scripted audio GI programme was selected for being soothing and versatile Researchers suggested that the interventions could be combined in a future study to investigate synergistic effects

Giacobbi et al. (2015)	To review the effects of GI for adults with arthritis and other rheumatic diseases	Systematic review of seven studies representing participants (n=287) completing the interventions/control subjects	Pre- and post-testing of a range of outcome measures, including pain, anxiety, depression and QoL	All studies except one reported significant improvements in outcomes	GI scripts were via audio recordings Intervention varied between 1 and 16 sessions
Lee, Kim and Yu (2013)	To evaluate the effects of GI on stress and fatigue in patients undergoing radioactive iodine therapy for thyroid cancer	RCT (n=84), 44 in the experimental group and 40 for the control group	Global Assessment of Recent Stress, Revised Piper Fatigue Scale and Heart Rate variability at 3 points during the five-week study	The first 4 titles were the texts that had the most influence on the origins of the HEARTS Process. Other texts made a useful contribution as the different elements emerged.	CD included imagining a peaceful scene and the sound of waterfalls with encouragement to recall the smell of roses Patients were reminded to practise GI by text daily and by telephone call weekly

cont.

Study	Objective	Design	Outcome measures	Results	Comments on the intervention(s)
King (2010)	To review and summarise studies performed from 2001–08, which included GI for cancer pain	Electronic databases were searched using keywords: cancer, pain and GI Five studies (n=287) satisfied the criteria	Most included numerical pain scales 0–10 scoring and analgesic usage, with some measuring anxiety and mood measures scores	Most studies reported some benefit from the interventions, but the numbers of participants were small The reviewer was cautious about recommended GI for pain relief The reviewer was critical of the GI scripts in that they did not take account of diverse populations	All studies used audiotapes, some provided face-to-face short sessions of GI and PMR training GI scripts mostly focused on positive mood and pleasant imagery, supplemented by PMR instructions One suggested glove anaesthesia The reviewer suggested patients should be allowed to create their own place or image of relaxation and peacefulness

| Menzies, Taylor and Bourguignon (2006) | To evaluate the effects of six weeks of GI on pain level, functional status and self-efficacy for adults with fibromyalgia and to explore the dose-response effect of GI use on outcomes | Longitudinal, prospective, two-group RCT (*n*=48) | Short-Form McGill Pain Questionnaire (SF-MPQ), Arthritis Self-Efficacy Scale (ASES) and Fibromyalgia Impact Questionnaire (FIQ), at baseline, 6 and 10 weeks, and submitted frequency of use report forms | FIQ scores decreased over time in the GI group compared with the usual care group

Ratings of self-efficacy for managing pain and other symptoms also increased significantly over time in the GI group compared with the usual care group

Pain as measured did not change over time or by group

Imagery dosage was not significant | Three GI audio recordings focused on breathing, pleasant scenarios and feelings of wellbeing – suggestions were made to be creative with GI

Participants were encouraged to use the GI recordings daily

Small sample with variable pain and use of analgesics |

Chapter 6

TEXTURES AND HANDS-ON

KEYWORDS

Hands-on; textures; interface; Library of Strokes; intuition; massage

INTRODUCTION

This chapter begins by exploring the role of textures as an integral and important component for the Hands-on work. This is followed by an overview of the Library of Strokes, which is the foundation of the HEARTS treatment and provides the therapeutic use of touch (Carter 2006). The combination of touch and textures is the unique base for the demonstration of empathy, compassion and connection, which, in practice, bring HEARTS alive. A description of the Library of Strokes offers ways of using kind, well-intentioned touch, and focuses on working through different textures. Case studies are provided to illustrate the work in various settings, and recommendations are made for introducing and integrating HEARTS in the workplace. A brief comparison is made between the practice of HEARTS and massage towards the end of the chapter.

TEXTURES

Using well-intentioned touch through a fabric is fundamental to the HEARTS Process. The Hands-on touch work is always carried out through a texture, such as a soft blanket, a warm towel or the patient's own clothes, such as a dressing gown or shawl. In contrast to massage, a lubricant such as oil or cream is not used. Working through a fabric can provide a soothing and welcome interface between the therapist and patient. As textures have a fundamental role to play in HEARTS, it may be helpful to remind ourselves of the skin as 'a sensory canvas' on which the hands, working as 'brushes', can 'paint their art'.

Sanderson, Harrison and Price (1991) have described how using different textures for sensory stimulation can play an important role in the rehabilitation of young adults with learning difficulties. Using the principles that underlie the process of sensory stimulation, it was decided that instead of regarding dressing gowns, blankets and duvets as a hindrance, textures could be used to enhance the sensory experience of the Hands-on work. It is advantageous that the patient does not need to undress to receive the therapy, and covering a patient can increase the access and availability of touch for particularly vulnerable patients.

Before considering the benefits of textures, we need to address issues of hygiene and infection control. Working through the patient's own linen and clothing is important so we do not introduce the risks of cross-infection. The shedding of skin cells can be a medium for contamination when skin is disturbed, although placing a cloth fabric over a patient does afford a reduction in skin contact. Importantly, hand washing and the use of alcohol hand rubs are important when working with patients and carers in any care setting.

Textures may hold memories that can be used as an anchor for future treatments and comfort. A pivotal case study that illustrates this concept involves a knitted 'rainbow' blanket, which was provided by a volunteer in an elderly care setting.

Case study 6.1. Pleasant memories of a special blanket

Bridget was a resident in a care home. The knitted fabric reminded Bridget of her 'special' blanket that had been crocheted by her mother when Bridget was a small child. Bridget would cuddle the blanket while her mother told her bedtime stories, and it went with her everywhere. The therapist asked, 'Where would you like me to place the blanket, Bridget, while I gently work on your shoulders, arms and legs?' Bridget said she would like the blanket placed over her chest and up to her chin. After 10 minutes, she snuggled further into the blanket and drifted off to sleep. Bridget requested that the blanket be placed on her chest every night, saying it helped her to remember her mother and the bedtime stories.

SOME BENEFITS OF WORKING THROUGH TEXTURES

Depending on the environment, a patient can be covered with a fabric that may promote feelings of security or a recall of nurturing memories from childhood. The patient may be wrapped in, or covered with, a soft blanket, which may also suggest memories of affection, caring and closeness. Additionally, some people have a special attachment to a particular blanket or shawl, which is of emotional significance. Restoring a link between the fabric and something with which the patient has a positive emotional attachment may assist in accessing a pleasant state of calm.

A major benefit of using textures is that patients with limited coordination, and those who have body image concerns, do not have to remove clothing. We can also work through a patient's existing clothing or bedclothes, so the patient need not feel anxious about too much intimacy (in-to-me-see). For patients who are wary about the degree of intimacy in massage, where cream or oil is applied directly to the skin, the additional 'layer' of cover can offer an enhanced sense of boundary. Every time the therapist is able to change the texture through which s/he works, the patient will receive a different sensory experience, and the therapist can vary the Library of Strokes accordingly (see below).

As well as the 'feeling of the fabric' we may also need to consider the weight of bedcovers and how they are placed. If HEARTS is given through existing bedclothes, it is likely that more covering will not be necessary as it could add unnecessary weight. However, if the skin is bare, or where the hands and arms are exposed above the bedcovers, it may be pleasant to put a small towel or lightweight blanket over this area, rather than working with skin-to-skin contact.

Once the texture is in place, the focus of the treatment becomes the practice of the touch work. McFarland (1988) describes what happens when touch begins. He advises, 'Place a hand upon a body and, in that very instant, that body is placed upon your hand, each simultaneously transmitting and receiving in a continuous process of shaping and reshaping and responding to each others input' (p.107). The Hands-on work is regarded as a two-way process, with therapists bringing their touch skills and their intention to help; the patient responds by engaging with the process and responding to the therapeutic process. The quality of the Hands-on work is dependent on the therapist being present in the moment, continuously being aware of how his/her hands are connecting, sensing and listening, while observing the responses of the patient (Cawthorn 2006).

LIBRARY OF STROKES

The Library of Strokes may be defined as 'different ways of touching someone with an aim of facilitating a calming or relaxing experience' (Carter 2017, p.171). The word 'library' implies that there is a miscellany of 'strokes' that the therapist could use. In addition to promoting calm and relaxation, the aim of the strokes is to create feelings of wellbeing and being cared for. There is no prescriptive way of using any of the strokes; it is up to the therapist to choose which of the strokes would be of optimum help for patient. Of course, a patient can be consulted about personal preferences, and this can be helpful in building empathy and trust.

Five core ways of using touch that form the focus of the HEARTS Process are described below. All of the strokes can be varied by the rhythm, pressure, speed and the amount of time for which each stroke is used. One exception is 'therapeutic holding', which is still and calming. However, the outcome can be affected by the degree of pressure applied and the amount of time the therapist spends 'holding' a part of the body, such as the feet, knees or hands. In HEARTS, the process of touching is one of creativity, where the therapist can 'tune in' to the patient and in turn, the patient can 'tune in' to the therapist's touch. In subsequent treatments, the patient may want to be more involved in designing his/her HEARTS session. Giving the patient choices is a very rewarding way of working, and on many occasions patients have enjoyed the option of engaging with the therapist and the treatment. The strokes described below are not finite, and it is likely that once a therapist is fully acquainted with the principles of HEARTS, s/he will want to bring in his/her own ideas and techniques that s/he particularly likes to use.

1. The strokedown

Using rhythmic stroking to work through textures is one of the most useful techniques in HEARTS. Maintaining a rhythm is the key to using the strokedown for optimum effect.

Basically, the strokedown is a gentle and rhythmic stroking in longitudinal and circular movements, possibly through a warm towel or other suitable fabric. However, we need to remember that when we are working through fabric, the stroking movements have to be adapted to accommodate the texture – it may be rough, smooth, silky, velvety... This is why it may be helpful to refrain from thinking of our work as 'massage through clothes or covers' and to consider the stroking and the other movements simply as what they are. The aim of promoting calm and relaxation remains a priority, but the primary contact is through the fabric; we do not have the same 'grip or slide' as when an oil or cream is used directly on the skin (see Chapter 3). The texture of the fabric and the friction (which moving hands will encounter) do not allow for heavy pressure. If there is too much pressure, the fabric may wrinkle and friction will be experienced through the therapist's hands; too much pressure will be uncomfortable for both the patient and the therapist.

Trying out the hand as a unit

When working through fabric, it is helpful for the hand to work as a single unit, as described in Chapter 3. Sometimes, the therapist will want to spread the thumb away from the hand; in this position the hands may want to grip, especially when working on an arm or a leg. Keeping the thumb and hand together enables the hand to work as a whole and offers a completely different experience (see Figures 6.1 and 6.2).

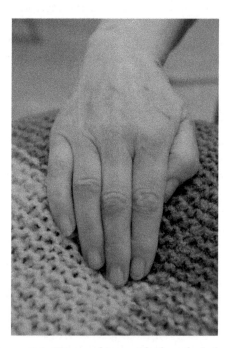

Figure 6.1. Try stroking with the whole hand

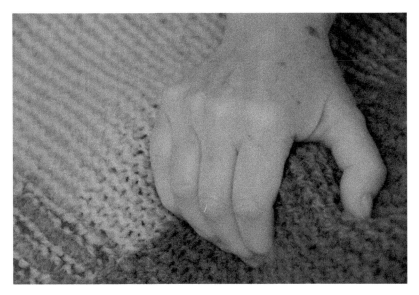

*Figure 6.2. Compare with stroking with the
thumb separate from the fingers, and notice the difference*

Try this for yourself on one of your own arms.

1. Keeping your thumb in contact with the rest of your hand, stroke upwards from your wrist to your shoulder slowly and lightly, and then let your hand slide back to its start point using light touch, maybe using your fingertips on the downward stroke.

2. Now separate your thumb from the rest of your hand as though you were going to stroke your arm with the hand in this position. (You may need to bend your arm.) Repeat the same movement. It is likely that you will find it harder to do; the thumb may want the whole hand to adopt a grip on the arm. The hand is very effective when it is used as a total unit, and it is also free of any tension that is promoted by gripping.

An example of how textures and the 'strokedown' can be used effectively is described in Case study 6.2.

Case study 6.2. Touch to ease an isolated patient

The therapist was asked to see a patient, Millie, who was due to leave hospital to be admitted to a hospice. She was facing a long journey, and the therapist found her sitting alone, on a chair near the bed, still wearing her white night clothes and a white dressing gown. The curtains were drawn around the bed and the patient looked very down, pale and isolated. After explaining how HEARTS worked and gaining consent, the therapist put a small towel around the patient's shoulders and used a combination of stroking movements and fingertip brushing (described below). She was only able to work on the patient's arms with some gentle work on the shoulders and upper back due to limited space. After a few minutes, a relative arrived and the patient signalled her relative away. The treatment took around 10 minutes, during which time colour came back into the patient's face, and her posture altered; it was more open and the patient seemed to sit taller on the chair. The patient said, 'I don't know what you've done, but I feel so much better than when you came in.'

2. Adapted palming

Just as effleurage is the stroke that is normally used to begin a Swedish massage treatment, palming is the stroke that is normally used to begin a session of shiatsu and Thai massage. Both these therapies are carried out through clothing, or in the case of shiatsu, the patient could be covered with a cotton sheet or cloth. Palming could be described as the reverse of the strokedown – the palms of the hands do not slide and the experience is one of achieving a 'still and gentle depth'. The technique has been adapted so that it is suitable for use with vulnerable patients. The whole of the hand is involved, although the palms have the major role. Adapted palming is suitable for large areas such as the back and areas where there is some muscle depth, such as on the forearms and thighs.

In HEARTS, the action is one of letting the hands 'sink into the tissue' slowly and alternately. The minimum of pressure is applied so the tissue 'lets you in' rather than the therapist deliberately applying what s/he thinks is the appropriate pressure for the patient. The application of achieving 'a gentle depth' offers an experience of security, stillness and 'grounding', especially when it is carried out slowly and gently. As palming in this context is slow, it is essential to give the patient time to absorb the sensation from the gentle pressures and an alternating pattern of synchronised hand movements.

Palming can be likened to the movements of a cat, often purring contentedly, as it gently moves from one paw to the other in a similar seesaw manner.

Practising the seesaw movement on your thighs

To practise the seesaw movement, follow these steps:

1. Sit comfortably and rest one hand on each thigh.

2. Start with your dominant hand by letting the hand sink into the soft tissue, while the other hand rests gently on the other thigh.

3. Shift the attention to the other hand; allow this second hand to sink into the soft tissue of the thigh, while lightening the touch of the dominant hand.

4. Repeat steps 2 and 3 in a sequence of five times, to experience the transfer of weight, and to notice your hands creating a rhythmic seesaw movement.

By using the hands alternately, a large surface area of the body can be covered. The weight transference will need to be applied as the hands continue to move, so covering the area on which the therapist is working. This is a slow, grounding movement, allowing time for the patient to experience the gentle 'pressure' of the hands sinking into the tissues. I suggest practising a few times to establish the 'sink and release rhythm' and once achieved, to then explore ways of covering an area.

Practising palming (see Figures 6.3–6.6)

A friend's back is a useful place to practise with your friend lying supine. (If no one is available, you can practise on soft furniture, such as a chair arm, a sofa or a bed. If you are practising on some soft furniture, decide a point A, which is your start point, and your hands will move to point B, which is further along the arm or the cushions.)

The following sequence is for learning the rhythm with alternating 'pressures'. The process starts at the shoulders and the hands will move pedad (which means towards the feet).

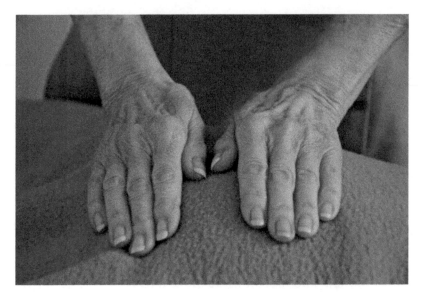

Figure 6.3. Step 1: Place your hands side by side with the right hand resting on the shoulder blade and the left hand next to it

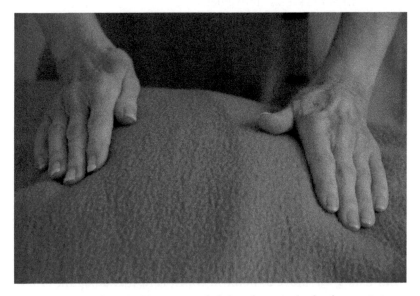

Figure 6.4. Step 2: Move your left hand towards the feet so it is approximately one width of your hand away from the right hand. Apply gentle pressure with the left hand that has just moved

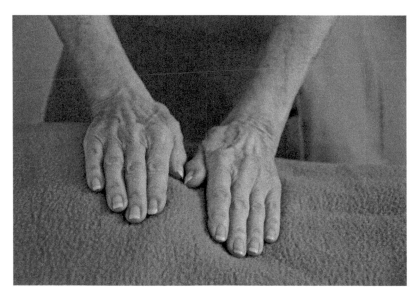

Figure 6.5. Step 3: Bring the right hand towards the feet to join the left hand. Release the pressure with the left hand and apply the sinking pressure with the hand you have just moved

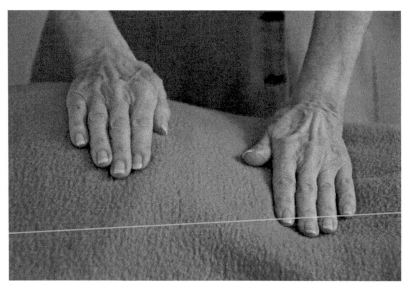

Figure 6.6. Step 4: As you apply pressure with the right hand, move the left hand towards the feet (as you did in Step 1) and apply gentle pressure once again

These four steps form the sequence and it is much easier to do than to describe. At first you may find your hands will find it easier to work in a straight line, but as you become more familiar with the rhythm and the alternating pressures, you will find that your hands will become more adapted to the contours of the patient's body.

It is helpful if the patient is allowed time to experience the value of this touch technique, so it needs to be slow and calming; pauses or moving strokes can be introduced where necessary. This approach is particularly pleasant to receive using a massage chair, or where the patient is supported by pillows while leaning against a bed, a couch or a table. If the patient is supine it can be easily applied to the upper arms and thighs. The technique is less suitable where there may be little muscle or fluid retention. Therapeutic holding can be used as a substitute in these areas if necessary. It is more difficult to apply this technique if the patient is lying in the middle of a bed due to the posture needed by the therapist to apply the palming easily and effectively. It may be more beneficial to choose another option or to ask for help in finding the optimum position for the patient. (Never attempt to move a patient on your own, for both your own safety and that of the patient.)

3. Fingertip brushing

Most of us enjoy the sensation of someone raking their fingers down our backs. The fingertips can be used in many ways. It is a lovely way to complete a treatment or to contrast the sensations experienced through the stroking movements (strokedown) or palming. Using the fingertips can be a pleasant interlude between other techniques. It is likely that the patient will be in a supine position and the fingertips can be used on small areas, or longer strokes can applied such as finger brushing on the legs, the arms, or brushing the whole body from head to toe.

4. Therapeutic holding

The aim of therapeutic holding is to promote a state of calm and stillness. Therapeutic holding is a contrast to both the strokedown and adapted palming. It may be possible to use therapeutic holding at the start or end of the treatment, as well as at appropriate times during the session.

Many therapies already use these this approach, which is often carried out by resting the hands on a patient's head or feet at the beginning or the end of a treatment. In HEARTS, the purpose of therapeutic holding is to let the patient know you are there, to create an interlude between the different strokes you have chosen to use, and/or to promote a sense of security. It is also used to promote the release of tension where there has been pain that may have been due to a holding pattern.

Therapists often ask about a precise hand position that offers the optimum way of 'holding'. Both therapist and patient are unique individuals, with different sizes and shapes of hand of the giver, and different shapes and sizes of different areas of the body of the receiver. A practical way to find an 'optimum' position is to think of your hands as jigsaw puzzle pieces. Place them on the body, either on a flat area, or cupping an area such as a joint. When the hands are in the 'optimum' position for the individual, it is likely that you will experience a 'comfortable fit', just like two jigsaw puzzle pieces that match. It may be helpful to ask the patient for some feedback. S/he may say something like, 'Just move your hand to the outside a bit' and as soon as your hands are in the right place, the patient will say, 'That's it, it's lovely!' and you, too, will feel that your hands are in the optimum place. The patient may want to hold your hands and move them to an optimum position. Once this 'fit' is obtained, a process called 'melding' may be experienced. Melding occurs where heat is generated and your hands and the patient's tissues feel as though they are being 'held' together; often it is difficult to tell the difference where the interface between the two exists. Therapeutic holding can also promote a profound state of relaxation and 'connection' between therapist and patient.

Another way of using therapeutic holding is to apply it in a sequence, so it can be used over the whole body. Therapeutic holding is applied to the use of 'landmarks' or a 'body map', which are specific locations on the body. A useful sequence for landmarking is to put your hands on the feet, then the ankles, the front of the lower legs, the outside of the thighs, the hips, the shoulders, the upper arms, the lower arms, the hands and the wrists and where accessible, the patient's head. It may not be necessary or desirable to work on every location in a single treatment; the therapist can vary the approach as s/he chooses.

Sometimes therapists like to begin a treatment at the patient's head. If the patient is lying on a couch, this is easy to do, but it may not be possible if the person is in a bed, in which case, the therapist needs to take into account his/her own posture as there are some areas that will not be possible to reach. Another issue to consider is that it might be useful to begin the session where the patient can see you. If you stand behind the patient, s/he may want to keep his/her eyes open so s/he can see where you are, until s/he understands how the process works.

5. Breeze strokes

Initially a hand-held fan, similar to those used in the East, was used to create air movement along the body as a finishing movement. However, this was not the most practical of approaches and 'breeze strokes' were added at a later date, replacing the original idea of using a hand-held fan. Breeze strokes can be introduced as the physical strokes get lighter and lighter until the therapist is stroking in an area that is a short distance away from the body (possibly about 2 cm or half an inch). These strokes are not concerned with 'channelling' energy or chi, or balancing the aura... The purpose is to seek to be non-invasive and create flow, sometimes warmth, and even a sensation of gentle care around an area.

Combining the above

The ways in which you can use the above may be varied by:

- The total time that is available for Hands-on work – this may influence your aim and how you use the Library of Strokes.

- The speed(s) at which you choose to work.

- The pressure that you feel is the optimum to use.

- The textures through which the strokes are applied.

- The regularity of the rhythm.

- The amount of therapeutic holding introduced.

- The way in which the therapist's hands are used. (Forearms may also be used gently, especially on areas such as the patient's back.)

- Whether HEARTS is used on its own or as an integral part of a complementary therapy.

In using HEARTS there is no set pattern for using the Hands-on approaches described above. What is important is your intention and applying the movements in a way that is suitable for the patient. Often, when we begin our journey in complementary therapies, we learn a set routine on which we will be assessed for a qualification. However, it is likely that as we become more experienced, we will want to deviate from this initial routine. Some of the pleasures and challenges for a therapist arise in designing an individual treatment that is 'in the moment' for a patient.

TWO THERAPISTS, ONE PATIENT

Another variation that can be helpful and enjoyable for all concerned is for two people to work on one patient at the same time. One takes the role of lead therapist, while the other acts as the 'follower', and mirrors approximately how the lead therapist is working. As the two therapists will be working on different areas of the body, matching rhythm and speed are important. The therapists can work opposite each other on the upper and lower parts of the body, or they can work longitudinally, so each works either side of the body. Another option is for one therapist to hold an agreed part of the body, such as the feet, hands or head, while the other does gentle stroking movements (see Figures 6.7 and 6.8).

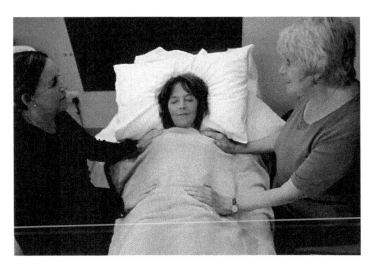

Figure 6.7. Therapists can work opposite each other...

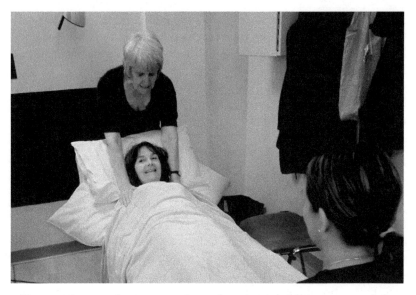

Figure 6.8. ...or they can work on the upper and lower areas of the body. This can be an enjoyable experience for all concerned

It is also helpful to agree how you will start and end the treatment. One of the most pleasant ways is for the lead therapist to start and for the 'follower' to join in (having agreed this with the patient before the treatment starts). Similarly, at the end of the treatment the follower can find a way to end his/her role with the lead therapist concluding the treatment.

This method is useful when teaching carers as the carer can work alongside the therapist. It also means that more than one family member can work on the patient at the same time (see Chapter 11).

HEARTS AND THE SENSITIVITY OF THE SKIN

Some healthcare professionals (and therapists) may not believe that the human sensory system is sensitive enough to be stimulated through a duvet or through several blankets, but utilising gentle pressures through a duvet for someone who is very anxious can help to provide a sense of increased control and security (see Case study 6.3).

Case study 6.3. The comfort of a duvet during the night

Elsie, aged 75, had colon cancer with advanced metastatic spread. She was spending a few days in a hospice for respite care. At 3am she decided she wanted to use the bathroom, and on the way back to bed she fell and was very shaken by the experience. Once she was back in bed, she begged the nurses not to leave her. One of the nurses deliberately drew attention to the duvet with which Elsie was covered. Then she started to do gentle pressures through the duvet, asking Elsie to feel her hands working though the duvet. Slowly, Elsie began to calm, and after a few minutes she drifted into sleep and slept for the rest of the night.

THE DIFFERENCE BETWEEN HEARTS AND MASSAGE

Table 6.1 briefly outlines the main differences between HEARTS and massage. HEARTS can be integrated into a massage treatment at the beginning or end of the massage and may be used as an interlude during the massage once agreed with the patient (see Chapter 3).

Table 6.1. Some differences between HEARTS and massage

HEARTS	Massage
Light Hands-on contact	Soft tissue work
Contact through fabric/texture	Mostly skin-to-skin contact
Includes integrated imagery	Conversation minimal
No lubricant	Lubricant used (oil or cream)
Calming and soothing	Primarily soft tissue release
Library of Strokes	Effleurage, petrissage, tapotement
Music is chosen as an integrated part of the treatment	Music is used as background and is often chosen by the therapist
Can be integrated into other therapy treatments	Primary treatment

RECOMMENDATIONS

- Be prepared to explain the touch and texture components of HEARTS and how they might differ from traditional massage to patients, carers and healthcare professionals.

- It may be helpful to have a leaflet about touch and textures available and to be able to explain the process of self-soothing and recalling of the treatment to a patient.

- Always be prepared to work with materials/textiles that are readily available in your work environment, mindful of infection control, patient comfort and ideally patient preference.

- Rehearse the use of textures and the Library of Strokes with family, friends and colleagues who can offer you feedback.

SUMMARY

This chapter has covered the fundamental principles of using touch and textures within the HEARTS Process. The value of working through textures and with suitable touch techniques has been explained. The Library of Strokes has been described and case studies have been used to illustrate some of the principles of HEARTS. The characteristics of HEARTS and massage have been described in a table as a follow-on to Chapter 3. Some recommendations have been made concerning practising HEARTS and its integration into the workplace.

Chapter 7

SOUND

KEYWORDS
music; human voice; commentary; invitational language;
person-centred guided imagery (PCGI); colour

INTRODUCTION

Music is possibly the most common use of sound in complementary therapy sessions, and this chapter explores some of the therapeutic effects of the use of background music. Central to the chapter is discussion of a variety of options for integrating the human voice into the HEARTS process; the aim is to integrate simplified 'person-centred guided imagery' (PCGI) into the touch work. Learning to use one's own unique voice therapeutically can present both challenges and developmental opportunities for the therapist. Challenges are identified and suggestions made to assist therapists in developing confidence and expertise in this component of HEARTS. Simplicity is the key to the resourceful use of the voice, but keeping the words and sentences 'simple' does not detract from their contribution to the therapeutic process. This chapter should be read with reference to Chapter 5 on Relaxation and Chapter 8 on Aromas, where a further approach to devising PCGI is described.

THE POTENTIAL ROLE OF MUSIC

There are many ways in which therapists use background music to help promote a state of calm, and in many situations this works well. However, it also needs to be acknowledged that some therapists will automatically put on their favourite CD as a comforting ritual to support their work. Sometimes the patient welcomes this and may request details of the music for home use. Patients may also welcome the therapist's chosen music as a pleasant 'addition' to the treatment. Some patients are uncomfortable with silence and music helps to 'fill the space', thus aiding calm or relaxation. Music that is both familiar and holds positive memories can act as a source of 'helpful focus' for the mind, bringing some structure and security to the session. For those living with dementia, research and anecdotal evidence report that a familiar piece of music can assist in a spontaneous recall of memories. This may facilitate the singing of a song or the recalling of dance moves, resulting in greater interaction with carers and the wider world (Arroyo-Anlló, Díaz and Gil 2013) (see Chapter 10).

Much of the research concerned with the contribution that music can make in cancer care is focused on the benefits of music therapy; treatments are tailored to individuals, their choices and their needs. Bro *et al.* (2017) conducted a systematic review of the use of music with adult patients who had cancer. The review included 25 randomised controlled trials that met the criteria for a review. They found that the most effective mode of music intervention appeared to be passive listening to self-selected, recorded music. While acknowledging that the quality of the research reviewed was rated from low to very low, they concluded that the use of music can reduce anxiety, pain and low mood in this target group. Rosetti *et al.* (2017) conducted a survey to evaluate the impact of music therapy on anxiety and distress during medical procedures in patients who were newly diagnosed with head and neck or breast cancers ($n=78$). There were two groups of equal numbers in the study. One group received an individual consultation with a music therapist who helped the patient make his/her own choice of music, which was played during medical procedures. The second group did not receive a consultation and no music was played. In the group that received music during the procedures, there was a significant lowering of anxiety and distress scores.

In clinical settings, music could be played in a private room, but in an open area, headphones would be necessary so as not to disturb other patients. This makes interaction between the therapist and patient difficult and also limits access to the head and face. Dependency on music and supporting technology may prevent spontaneous provision of an intervention in complex situations. If music is available, then ideally its use should be of the patient's choice. There should at least be some options in place, so that the patient can agree a sound level and cessation at any point. However, the human voice is an asset that we have with us at all times, wherever the patient is, and whatever the reason for an intervention.

WHY USE YOUR OWN VOICE?

The brain is 'hardwired' to 'tune into' the human voice, with the sound of our mother's heart beat, breathing, digestion and voice among our first experiences of sound in the womb. There is evidence that babies can hear music, voices and other sounds in the womb (Moon and Fifer 2000). Even as adults, a comforting voice can help, recalling positive childhood memories of caring and being 'looked after', which can ease and soothe us in moments of distress.

During a HEARTS session, the therapist's voice can be used as a resource to help calm the patient at the beginning of the treatment, to assist if the patient becomes restless, or at the end of the treatment to offer a calm conclusion. The patient may retain your voice in his/her memory long after the session is over; it can continue to travel with him/her, and be available as a resource at any time.

SOME CHALLENGES AND SOLUTIONS OF USING YOUR VOICE

There maybe a reluctance and lack of familiarity when working therapeutically with the voice; its use may be associated with counselling, hypnotherapy or psychotherapy. In the context of HEARTS, challenges for the therapist may originate from the following. Some solutions are suggested in the text.

1. Hearing the sound of my own voice

When we hear external sounds, the vibrations travel externally to the outer ear (the pinna); from there, the vibrations travel to the cochlea in the inner ear, and then on to the brain, where interpretation of the sound takes place. A therapist may or may not like hearing the 'sound of his/her own voice'. As our voice vibrations are generated internally, the sound waves also travel through the bones of the head and into the inner ear, so, in effect, we are hearing ourselves from two different directions, internally and externally. The sound of our own voice is amplified by bone, which changes the frequency of the sound waves, so sound appears louder than it would normally be. When we hear a recording of our own voice we may be surprised, or even embarrassed, by the way it sounds.

Suggestion: If we can listen purposefully to our voice, we can start to make changes – for example, slowing down words, lowering the tone of the voice and including pauses.

2. Using two therapeutic approaches at the same time

The therapist is probably more familiar with using touch as a single therapy in the course of his/her everyday practice. The potential for incorporating the resourceful use of the human voice as part of a treatment may not have been explored. When you read a story to a child, your pace and tone change as you take note of full stops and speech marks, and what is happening with the characters in the story. If we were to demonstrate making a cup of tea, we would use a verbal commentary to support our actions with the tea, the teapot and the kettle. Giving a commentary in HEARTS is akin to these processes; you simply engage the patient by 'telling a story' about what your hands are doing.

The tone of your voice and the words need to be in emotional 'harmony' or 'match' so they are congruent with your intention. If words such as 'relax' or 'calm' are spoken with a short vowel and a harsh tone, the words can sound like a command. As a result, the tone and words may be perceived to be discordant with the aims of the treatment.

Suggestion: Remembering to breathe is an important part of the process – taking a slow outbreath will help to pace your delivery and will also help to soften the tone.

3. Being observed and listened to by others

It can be quite a daunting prospect for a therapist if s/he knows that others are taking an interest in how s/he is working with the patient, especially if the sound of a voice is coming from behind a curtain. We are all naturally curious, and, if the sounds are comforting and calming, it is likely that others may wish for the soothing effect. Most healthcare professionals will be paying attention to using their professional skills in providing patient care, and it is more likely that they will be more interested in the therapist's approach, rather than being judgemental.

Suggestion: If you are on a ward where you can be either overheard by other patients or observed by a carer, use positive self-talk. Welcome the opportunity to extend the relaxation to the environment surrounding the patient as part of your overall intention for the session. Bystanders, such as healthcare staff and carers, will soon tell you how calming it is just watching and listening to you, often saying they would like to swap places, so that they, too, could have the same experience (see Chapter 12).

4. Running out of something to say...
saying less may be more

In HEARTS, there are suggested frameworks for using the voice that can be linked to how the therapist is working at the time. Much of the content that the therapist offers verbally to the patient is framed in either a commentary or a 'narrative' of the patient's own construction (see Chapter 8). In the case of a commentary, there are prompts implicit in the way the hands are being used. If you are concerned about running out of words, one technique is to pause, and then repeat the same sentence in a slightly different way. Alternatively, you could tell the patient that just for a few moments, you are going to take a break from using your voice, so that the patient can focus on the Hands-on work, suggesting that the patient may like to focus on the sensations that s/he is experiencing from the stroking or therapeutic holding. Trusting in the process may sound glib, but running out of words may be a signal to slow down and let your hands to do the work for a short time.

Suggestion: Again, remember to breathe. A focused inbreath, followed by a soft sigh with a longer outbreath, may trigger a similar response in the patient.

5. I have an accent!

Sometimes a therapist will express concern that his/her voice, accent or tone is not suitable for this work. Given that we live in a multicultural society with our own unique histories, it may be that the words we commonly use may be less familiar to the patient. The rhythm, tone of voice and pacing of the words will convey the helpful intent behind the phrases we use, although the words may feel clumsy or inappropriate at the time.

Often, patients tell us that they appreciate a treatment being specially designed for them. Constructive feedback is usually concerned with a request for the therapist to slow the speed at which s/he speaks, rather than any criticism of the tone of the therapist's voice. There is no need for a therapist to look for a 'magical ingredient'. A calm voice in a slightly slower pace than normal will suffice.

Suggestion: Slow the delivery, emphasising some of the words and slightly elongating the vowels in words that carry your intention, such as caalm, sooothe, feeling at eease, etc.

6. Working with hearing difficulties

If the patient has a hearing impairment, you may need to work nearer to the patient's ear, at least initially; varying the volume, tone and rhythm is always useful. Non-verbal cues, such as smiling and 'kind eyes', can also affect how the emotional tone of the voice is carried. Aside from a patient relying on a hearing aid, s/he may prefer to lip read, as long as the therapist's face is in view.

Suggestion: Remember – using the voice in HEARTS is not a performance: it is a way of assisting a patient to experience calm, relaxation and to feel at ease.

All of the above 'challenges' can be overcome by acquiring some 'know-how' and then practising to refine skills and boost confidence. In addition to enhancing outcomes for patients, using the voice also assists the therapist in being fully present and focused. With practice, I believe that using the voice can become like 'knitting words together' without the need for a pattern.

The following comment was recently sent from a therapist who regularly practises HEARTS. It is typical of the comments from many other HEARTS therapists when they have been able to use voice work with patients:

> 'When I finished the HEARTS training, I loved the touch work, but wasn't happy with the using my voice. However, I pushed myself to use it regularly and I now find that it really enhances my other skills and I think it makes my treatments more effective. I love sharing the gift of stillness and relaxation with my patients.'

THREE SIMPLE APPROACHES FOR USING THE VOICE

Some suggestions for using the voice, working together with the Library of Strokes, are outlined below. These approaches are designed for simplicity and to complement the principles that underpin HEARTS. The principles of each approach can be varied to suit the individual patient's needs. All three approaches have a degree of 'patient involvement' implicit in the approach. A suitable contract must be agreed with the patient before treatment starts.

1. The commentary

Originally, the commentary was designed for patients who were particularly vulnerable and who wanted to be more at ease with the process of relaxation. It was the intention to use the hands and voice together so that the kinaesthetic and auditory senses were experienced synergistically and the patient could 'listen to a story' about how the therapist's hands were working. Any of the following methods may be used for helping a patient to self-soothe by recalling the touch sensations and the sound of the therapist's voice (see Chapter 5). As you read through the following, you may like to become aware of the invitational style of the language used. (For clarification, this has been written in italics.)

The process

1. Place your hands on the patient's ankles or on the front of the feet.

2. Invite the patient to bring his/her awareness to where your hands are placed, for example, '*I would like to invite you to become aware of my hands resting on your feet...*'

3. Invite the patient to 'become aware' of the 'landmarks'[1] as you work up the body in a sequence, physically putting your hands on the 'landmarks'. The easy 'landmarks' are the feet, ankles, knees, outer thighs (or the tops of thighs), hips, hands, wrists, arms, shoulders and under the neck and head. You could say something to the patient like '*...and now, you may like to become aware of my hands resting on your knees...and now let your attention drift to my hands resting gently on your hips – and you may like to notice, that, as you bring your awareness to where my hands are resting, that you may feel even more comfortable and more at ease...*' You can work through the 'landmarks'[2] in this manner, commenting on where your hands are placed and inviting the patient to 'become aware' or 'notice' where

---

1   You can start the Hands-on work at any place on the body.
2   There is no need to visit every single landmark; it would also be very monotonous to visit and comment on every one. Observe the patient's response and when they are relaxed, reduce or stop the use of your voice. See Case study 7.1, which demonstrates the use of this approach.

your hands are 'gently resting'. Additionally, you could say '*...and you may like to become aware as I gently stroke from the top of your shoulder...down through your upper arms...your elbows...into your forearms, down through your wrists, and now I am gently stroking the back of your hands from your wrists to your fingertips.*' This wording can be altered to be compatible with the person with whom you are working and the kind of touch you are using at the time.

Case study 7.1. Changing an attitude through experiencing HEARTS

Chris had advanced bowel cancer and was dubious about this 'touchy feely stuff'. Eventually he agreed to be referred for HEARTS, possibly to please the nursing staff. The therapist explained the process and started gentle palming and stroking work on Chris's left arm. Chris remained alert, looking at the ceiling, with a faint smile on his face. The therapist stopped the treatment and asked Chris to consent for the therapist to use her voice as a commentary. With consent obtained, she started by saying, 'Chris, you may like to become aware of my hands and the gentle pressure on your upper arms... And now as I am stroking slowly from your shoulders, all the way down to your fingertips, as I do this, you may become aware of the different sensations in your arms as my hands gently stroke from your shoulder, all the way down through your elbow...your lower arms...your wrists and your hands.' Chris's eyes remained open for a while, but his face was visibly more relaxed and he seemed to be listening. The therapist continued speaking in this way until she had repeated the commentary and touch work on both arms. By this time, Chris had closed his eyes and his breathing had altered. The therapist said, 'I am going to stop speaking, Chris, while I begin the gentle pressures we talked about. I will speak again when I am nearing the end of the treatment.' To conclude, the therapist said, 'I am resting my hands on the front of your feet, and I would like to invite you to notice how that feels, knowing that you can recall this experience at any time...and now I am going to complete our session by gently squeezing the sides of your feet.' Slowly, Chris opened his eyes and said, 'I take it all back...there's more to this than I thought.'

2. The comfort journey through the body

This approach was devised for patients who were more confident and who needed a brief 'introduction' to begin engaging with the Hands-on work. In the process outlined below the treatment starts at the feet. However, it could just as easily start on any part of the body such as the knees, hands or head, as requested by the patient.

1. Place your hands gently on the front of the feet or the ankles.

2. Suggest that the patient becomes aware of what it is like for him/her to have your hands in that position. Patients usually notice an experience of warmth, comfort or calm.

3. You may need to prompt; it is not uncommon for a patient to say, 'It's nice.' 'Nice' is sometimes referred to as a 'grateful word', but it does not represent any sensory experience. You may like to suggest, '...*my hands may feel warm... or you may find them calming...or soothing, or something else that is your own word*'. Usually, the patient will come up with a sensory 'resourceful' word. (The advantage of using the patient's own word is that s/he is already involved with the experience, and it is likely that the word will have some meaning for him/her.)

4. When the patient has identified a suitable sensory experience, such as calm or warmth, suggest that this pleasant feeling could travel through the patient's body – suggest the route, keeping the 'directions' in sequence and following the 'landmarks'. The hands can remain in one place throughout the 'sensory imagery', or you can use your hands and voice simultaneously to take the 'comfort feeling' through the body or to the places where it is needed.

5. Once the patient is accepting the relaxation process, the Hands-on work can begin.

An example of a patient's experience that illustrates this process is given in Case study 7.2.

Case study 7.2. Helping to reduce procedural anxiety

Asha had advanced ovarian cancer. Waiting for drainage of ascites, her stomach was feeling very distended and she was anxious about the procedure. The therapist was asked to see Asha, but she had limited time before she was due to go to the procedures unit. The therapist briefly explained how she may be able to help, and asked if she could put her hands on somewhere that Asha would find comfortable. Asha was happy to consent and replied, 'I love having my feet done.' Placing her hands on Asha's feet over the bed sheet, the therapist held them in one place for a few moments before asking Asha about how it felt. Asha said 'My feet feel lovely and cosy in your hands.' The therapist said, 'Now, I would like to invite you to take that cosy feeling upwards...through your lower legs and up to your knees. Now take the feeling up to your thighs...and into your hips... Now, once the cosy feeling has arrive...you may like to take that sensation into your tummy and lower back... Let it settle there...and...if there is anywhere else you where you would like that cosy feeling to travel, just let the sensation flow to that part of your body, where it might also be needed. I will sit by your side and gently hold your hips..., just using gentle pressures from your hips...down the outside of your thighs, through your knees, your lower legs and back to your feet.' Asha drifted into a doze and after a few minutes of stroking Asha's lower legs, the therapist told Asha that she was going to leave her resting and suggested that she may like to use the process during any clinical treatments as needed. The therapist left and she let the nurses know what she had provided. The following day Asha said she had used the image of the flow of cosiness throughout the procedure, and it was much easier than she thought it would be. Now, with the fluid drained, the discomfort had eased considerably.

3. Using colour as a resource

This approach was devised for patients who had requested an easy imagery technique that could be used when the therapist was not available. The patient can agree the 'feeling' s/he wants to promote with the therapist, but it is probably better if s/he doesn't tell the therapist her personal colour choice. As a therapist, there is an advantage to not knowing the patient's chosen colour(s); you cannot add your own experience of the patient's colour to the treatment.

Anecdotally, a patient insisted on telling the therapist that her chosen colour was a mix of black and pink. As these are the colours of a well-known sweet, the therapist had difficulty in not laughing as she imagined the black and pink sweets travelling round the body!

1. Ask the patient to think of a colour that represents one of the following: a feeling of comfort, or calm, or relaxation… or another word of the patient's choice.

2. When the patient has chosen his/her colour, agree a start point for where the colour will be introduced into the body, for example, the hands, head or feet. With your hands in contact with the start point, ask the patient to bring the colour into the body and let it travel to desired areas. The 'landmarks' can be used to track the movement of colour, bringing with it the chosen feeling.

Most patients like this approach, although a few might say it does not work for them. Some will change the colour for use in different parts of the body, and they need to know this is acceptable. One patient had a different colour for the left and right of the body; another had multiple colours that repeatedly changed. Our goal is not to impose any beliefs around colour – any colour(s) or even something neutral is good enough. Case study 7.3 illustrates this process of using colour.

Case study 7.3. Promoting quiet and restful sleep

Joyce came to an open relaxation group with a blood transfusion in progress. The previous night she had experienced a nightmare, and she wondered if there was anything that could help to reduce the chances of this happening again. The therapist offered to do some relaxation with Joyce that would involve touch work and colour. She asked Joyce to think of a colour that represented an opposite and welcome sensation to that of the distress. The therapist added that she did not need to know what the colour was – it was specially for Joyce's personal use. Joyce opted to rest on a massage couch and explained how she wanted the pillows arranged for maximum comfort. At Joyce's request, the therapist sat at Joyce's head, which was the start point for the colour to begin its journey round the body. The therapist asked Joyce to take her chosen colour around her body following a landmark sequence. The therapist completed the session with some Hands-on work and suggested that Joyce might like to recall the colour and the sequence whenever she felt the need. By using this approach, Joyce could recall her experience on the couch and was delighted to report a good night's sleep, with no recurrence of the nightmare.

RECOMMENDATIONS

- Rehearse – a good friend can be helpful as a 'model'. When you experiment with your voice, particularly with the rhythm and tone, do not be surprised if laughter occurs! Practise in short sessions and know what you want to achieve in each session – this will offer you a more focused use of time. It may help to practise a HEARTS commentary with a friend.

- Build up your own list of 'opening and closing words' based on invitational language and phrases which promote your intention; these can become part of your evolving tool box.

- Although I would recommend a person-centred approach where possible, sometimes the patient does not have the cognitive ability or the energy to want to participate. In such situations, a useful phrase is to say something like, 'How would it be if we did some team work?' or if s/he really can't participate, than use a method that you have tried and tested. It is still possible to monitor the patient's responses and ongoing consent.

- When a patient is poorly or fearful of the process, the simpler the sentences and words used, the easier it is for him/her to become engaged with the treatment. Sometimes it can be difficult to relate to long, complicated sentences that may have little relevance.

- Remember to bring a session to a conclusion rather than an abrupt end by slightly increasing the volume of the voice and its pace.

- A 'concluding signal' may be achieved by a gentle squeezing of the feet or hands or a stroke down the whole body. Additionally, you may like to suggest to the patient that s/he could recall the session and the sound of your voice when it would be helpful to do so.

- Listen to your patients' feedback and experience of HEARTS. Patients are our best teachers and can inform our developing practice.

SUMMARY

Music has been acknowledged as a useful resource for calming and eliminating silence with which some patients are uncomfortable. While acknowledging the initial challenges in developing skills in using your voice, it can become a useful and resourceful process. Some approaches to using the voice have been discussed. There are many rewards, especially as the therapist knows that s/he always has an extra resource wherever s/he is working. The principles and processes involved also help patients to develop an individual resource to help self-soothing by recalling the memory of the therapist's voice and the sensory experience of the touch work. It also helps to practise, and recommendations for developing voice skills have been given.

Chapter 8

AROMAS

KEYWORDS
olfaction; aromas; smell memory; person-centred guided
imagery (PCGI); essential oils; aromasticks

INTRODUCTION

There are two parts to this chapter – the first part describes the structure of the olfactory system and its relationship to the 'smell memory'. The potential for using the smell memory to involve patients in creating person-centred guided imagery (PCGI) sessions is explored, and case studies are used to illustrate how a personal narrative that has been developed from a sensory framework can be used to help a patient create his/her own 'story' for guided imagery (see Chapter 5). The second part focuses on the use of essential oils (EOs) and aromasticks in clinical settings, and includes recommendations for good practice.

ANATOMY AND PHYSIOLOGY OF THE OLFACTORY (SMELL) SYSTEM

The nose has two functions – one is to warm and filter incoming air, and the other is to house the first part of the olfactory system. At the top of the nose, on each side, is an olfactory lobe that is about the size of an almond. These two small lobes are covered in single-cell sensory receptors that are attached to a sensory nerve. Aromas are detected when airborne aromatic molecules stimulate these sensory receptor cells. However, the sensory receptors are of different shapes, and in order to stimulate the sensory nerves, an aromatic molecule has to match the shape of a sensory receptor. Once there is a 'lock and key' connection, a nerve stimulus is created. If aromatic molecules cannot find a receptor cell with which they can 'fit', the aroma cannot be detected. The scope for detecting different odours in humans is extraordinary. Bushdid *et al.* (2014) report that the human nose can detect at least 1 trillion different odours.

Interestingly, the olfactory cells are very sensitive and cease firing when over-stimulated.

The olfactory nerves lead from the olfactory lobes into part of the brain known as the olfactory bulb. The stimulus is then transmitted to the limbic system, which is the oldest part of the brain in evolutionary terms. Within the limbic system it is the amygdala and hippocampus that are responsible for the 'smell' memory and its link to the emotions.

Unless some form of physical impairment exists, most people have an 'olfactory memory'. Betts (1996) has stated that the sense of smell is very successful at recalling emotions and memories, both positive and negative. If the recall of an aromatic memory is positive, it is likely to initiate pleasant emotions and images for the patient. If the recall of the aroma was not pleasing, or is associated with an unhappy event, the reverse, negative reaction is likely to be generated.

ACCESSING A POSITIVE MEMORY THROUGH RECALLING AN AROMA USING PATIENT-CENTRED GUIDED IMAGERY

In Chapter 7, three approaches were suggested for using the voice. These were devised for their simplicity and compatibility with the Hands-on work. The following method of involving the patient in creating his/her own narrative is intended to be a brief intervention, probably around 5 minutes, plus the initial gathering of the information to make up the 'narrative'. The technique is not intended to generate a long, involved script; it serves to engage the patient in a pleasant mind activity that can be used at the beginning or end of a HEARTS session. For some patients this approach can become a useful method for self-soothing, which is described in Case study 8.1.

Aromatic recall is intended as an effective person-centred way of working. The method uses the patient's olfactory experience to help create the brief personal imagery session. Where the patient likes this approach s/he can continue to use it for self-soothing, for promoting sleep or during difficult procedures...or just for enjoyment.

Here are some examples of imagery created through recalling an aroma:

- A salty breeze at the seaside

- Eating key lime pie in a cafe when being on a weight loss diet

- Lemon trees in Greece

- Lavender and the patient's grandmother

- The smell of grandchildren

- Lilac blossom at an aunt's cottage in a small village

- Horse manure and the collecting ring at a horse show

- New-mown hay

- The aromas of spices at a festive event

- Hot buttered toast

- A Sunday roast.

Facilitating and recording the patient's narrative

1. Preparation: You will need some paper and pen/pencil for notes – it is unlikely that you will be able to remember all of the information that a patient gives to you. You will also need a basic knowledge of the use of sensory language; this will give you a framework to use at any time and anywhere (see Chapter 5).

2. Ask the patient to think of an aroma that generates a memory of an experience or an event that s/he feels comfortable to talk about; the scenario can be from the past or it can be an imagined event in the future. Another possibility is that an aroma can be recalled from everyday life in which the patient enjoys participating, for example, going for a favourite walk, being in a garden, a wood, or by the sea, having coffee with a friend, or playing with grandchildren.

3. Engaging the patient: Using the sensory framework outlined in Chapter 5, ask the patient about the content of their chosen scenario. (The gustatory sense (taste) is not always relevant – but it may be, depending on the individual's story, for example, the key lime pie.) Make some notes so that you can 'read' the patient's story back to him/her. Once you have the patient's 'narrative' in note form, agree with

the patient how s/he would like to receive it as part of the HEARTS session.

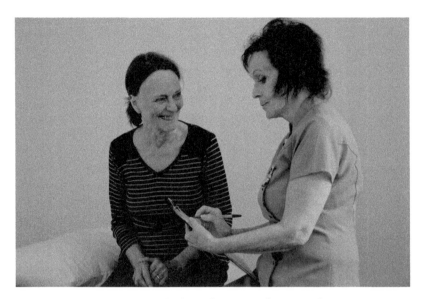

Figure 8.1. A clipboard or something similar is useful for recording the patient's story

There is a kind of reassuring intimacy for the patient if you place your hands on an agreed 'comfy' place such as the hands or feet while you relate the 'story'. You will need to put your notes where you can refer to them – ask the patient's permission to put the notes either on the bed or on the patient themselves. Case study 8.1 recounts the patient's 'narrative' that was told to the therapist. The sensory language referred to earlier in Chapter 5 is clearly evident.

Case study 8.1. Pleasant memories of a weekend

Jack was able to use his recall of a pleasant memory to assist sleep. He was not sleeping at night and was making up for lost sleep during the day. He also had a very enquiring mind and found it difficult to 'switch off'. As a result of being awake during the night, he did not want to engage with visitors and had to be woken for supportive treatments throughout the day. Apart from suggesting practical solutions such as drinking less caffeine late in the evening, the therapist suggested that Jack might find it helpful to direct his mind to something more relaxing. She set out to help him create an internal video of a pleasant memory with which he was comfortable, so that he could replay it whenever the 'other thoughts' became intrusive.

The therapist asked Jack about an aroma that he perceived to be 'a favourite smell' and that would be enjoyable and comfortable to work with. Immediately Jack said, 'Brandy and ginger'. He remembered a situation when he was courting and he was able to recall some happy evenings spent in a local pub in late summer. He could also recall the smell of cooking on the barbecue, and feel the chill in the air; he was able to recall how he and his girlfriend had walked along a path to a river where they could see the moon rise and the stars lighting up the dusky sky. Jack could feel his hand linked with his girlfriend's, and together they would listen to the sounds of the countryside in the evening, with the water rippling past them. Returning to the pub, he remembered 'seeing' them both, sitting in large, comfy armchairs, drinking their brandy and gingers, and chatting together. He could recall the sense of relaxation he felt as they sat together, their faces glowing from the warmth of the fire.

Jack's mood changed visibly from one of despondency to one of animation and being uplifted. The therapist used the material in the scenario as a relaxing introduction to the touch work in the Library of Strokes.

As Jack became more familiar with this method of recall, he began to think of an increasing number of pleasant and resourceful memories that were anchored with a significant aroma. Using the sensory framework he had learned from the therapist, he found that 'day dreaming' was a very pleasant way promote a feeling of calm.

4. Turning the patient's narrative into a 'story': Once a therapist has the narrative, in the patient's words, all s/he needs to do is to turn it into a story. An example of a patient's scenario as spoken by the therapist is detailed in Case study 8.2. In this case study, the therapist and patient (Carol) agreed to introduce the Library of Strokes after the imagery; the imagery was used to promote a sense of calm. The patient had talked about her garden and the smell of blossom on a few occasions, and she chose this scenario to create her PCGI session. Once again, as you read through it, notice how the sensory framework was used to create the experience. (The gustatory sense was not perceived to be relevant.) When you repeat the story back to the patient, I suggest that you start with the aroma to 'set the scene', then the other sensory images can be featured in any order. You will also notice the conversational style of delivery.

Case study 8.2. An example of PCGI in practice

Once the patient was comfortably positioned for the session, with the therapist resting her hands on the patient's knees, the therapist said: 'So, Carol, I would like to invite you to become aware of the beautiful smell of the blossom that you were telling me about...and let the aroma take you to a time when you were in your garden smelling the different kinds of blossom...and as you know there are other pleasant things to become aware of in your garden...you have told me about the colour of the flowers and the different kinds...the blue of the bluebells, the purple of the chives and the yellow of the early roses... You may notice a blackbird running across the lawn looking for worms...the sky is blue with white, fluffy clouds...and the aroma from the blossoms seems to pervade the whole garden... There are sounds that you can hear...someone's lawn mower from next door...and there is a thrush singing from the top of a cherry tree...it is lovely and uplifting to listen to the song... And there is sunshine... Feel the warmth of the sun on your shoulders as you walk down the yellow gravel path...hearing the crunch of the gravel and feeling the texture beneath your feet...And now, Carol, I am inviting you to become aware of the feeling that remembering the garden gives you, beginning to take that feeling round your body...'

...and it is here that the Library of Strokes could be introduced, for example, '...and now, Carol, I am going to let you enjoy the imagery that you have created, while I continue with the gentle strokes and pressures that you have told me you enjoy...'

5. When you are narrating the patient's story to them, remember that the experience belongs to the patient, and not to you. Don't tell the patient their story as though you are the first person, using 'I' all the way through the imagery. It is not your story, and to tell it in the first person may confuse the patient. It is essential that you dissociate from the patient's story by using the second person 'you', as demonstrated in Case study 8.2.

PCGI FOR SELF-SOOTHING

If a patient wants to continue to use this approach (as in Case study 8.1), it may be helpful to have some notes available that you can give to him/her for future reference. A second option, which may help to support some patients, is to make a live recording of the session, for which the therapist will need the patient's verbal agreement.

If there are any unwanted background noises, to acknowledge them in your 'retelling of the patient's story' will help to minimise their importance (see Chapter 5).

Sometimes therapists will want to record the scenario at a more convenient time 'to try to improve it' or to find a 'quieter place'. It is unlikely that the patient will expect the recording to be perfect; it is more likely that s/he will appreciate something that will help to recall the session, acting as a trigger of positive feelings. A separate recording does not have the same authenticity as when the patient is present. Making a new recording is time-consuming, and a perfectly quiet environment still cannot be guaranteed.

CONCERNS

Sometimes healthcare professionals who are involved in the patient's care may express concerns that recalling a memory could potentially upset the patient. I suggest that this is unlikely if the therapist explains that the invitational language used to guide the patient will be directed towards recalling a helpful/resourceful memory. There are options and the situation the patient chooses doesn't have to be a memory – it can be something current from everyday life. Additionally, it needs to be acknowledged that when patients are vulnerable, there can be everyday things, both in or outside of a HEARTS session, that may trigger emotions. The trigger could be seeing someone that reminds a patient of a loved one who has died, receiving bad news, detecting the familiar aroma of an aftershave or perfume, or even something that the therapist says can inadvertently trigger a memory. The key to supporting the patient is to suggest that it would be helpful if the 'smell memory' s/he chooses is something with which s/he feels comfortable. The therapist needs to make an initial judgement as to whether or not this method may be suitable for an individual.

METHODS OF USING ESSENTIAL OILS

Where essential oils (EOs) are integrated in the HEARTS Process, it is important that they should be prescribed by a qualified aromatherapist. EOs are more than a potentially pleasant smell; they are concentrated pharmaceutical agents. Their use requires knowledge, accountability and responsibility. Depending on the policies and procedures in the workplace, therapists and healthcare professionals who are not aromatherapists may be able to use the oils 'under the supervision' of a qualified aromatherapist who works in the same organisation.

It is assumed that an aromatherapist will gather information from the patient that will inform the choice and use of EOs that are prescribed for that individual. From reading therapists' case histories that relate to HEARTS, it seems that the most popular way of using EOs is to place between one and three drops of the chosen oil (or pre-prepared blend) on a tissue, a cotton wool ball or on the edge of a fabric cover. This could be a possible use of EOs if the method of use takes place in private practice, or where the patient is in his/her own room. The aroma can be deliberately 'anchored' during the treatment so that the patient can recall the pleasant experience associated with the treatment. However, in a clinical situation, such as a ward or where other patients are being treated, using this 'open' method of EOs presents some challenges, and may be unsuitable for that environment.

USING ESSENTIAL OILS IN A CLINICAL CONTEXT

Stringer and Donald (2011) describe some challenges concerning the use of essential oils in a hospital situation that would be helpful for therapists to consider. Where patients share their space with others, some patients may be experiencing chemotherapy-induced nausea and vomiting and/or have hypersensitivity to the aroma. EOs are very volatile and evaporate quickly, so there may be a risk to other individuals who are present in the vicinity. Some patients may experience sensitivity to the olfactory particles resulting in respiratory, skin and eye irritation. Additionally, the sense of smell is very individual, and an aroma that is loved by one patient may be perceived as totally unpleasant to another. An example of where a patient may have experienced totally unexpected symptoms in response to sweet orange oil is described in Case study 8.3.

Case study 8.3. An unexpected reaction to orange essential oil

Barry had come to the centre to see his key worker and to attend for a physiotherapy treatment. While sitting in the lounge, he became short of breath and started wheezing. The staff were very puzzled by his reaction and suggested that Barry should move to another area in the centre. As soon as he moved to a different area, the wheezing stopped. Barry reported that as he was sitting in the lounge, he became aware of the strong smell of oranges. On checking with the therapist who was using EOs at the time, she confirmed that she was using orange EO in a blend. It is possible that the orange EO could have been the irritant that caused Barry's respiratory problems.

THE USE OF AROMASTICKS

Aromasticks can be used to enhance a HEARTS treatment or to establish an 'anchor' that may help the patient to access the pleasant experience of the treatment when the therapist is no longer present. The patient may be experiencing emotions such as fear or anxiety, which can be ameliorated by inhaling from the aromastick.

For a therapist to set up using an aromastick with a patient can take time, so unless the patient has already been prescribed the oils and been shown how to use the aromastick, this may not be the best alternative in an emergency. However, if the patient already has an aromastick, it should be easy to integrate its use into a HEARTS treatment.

The structure of an aromastick

An aromastick consists of a cotton wick onto which the EOs are placed (see Figure 8.2). The wick is then placed inside a cylindrical plastic tube that is sealed at the base. At the top of the tube is a small, perforated opening through which the aroma can be inhaled. There is a protective outer cover that encloses the inner tube. The small opening at the top of the inner tube is an excellent way of enabling a patient to inhale an EOs blend in two ways. First, the use of the EOs blend by the patient is discreet; most of the EOs' molecules are contained inside the tube and the wick acts as a reservoir for continued use. Second, the small perforations help to prevent aromatic overload. This is where the patient likes the aroma so much that they continue to inhale it. An excess of an EOs blend can be overwhelming, which could make it unpleasant to use.

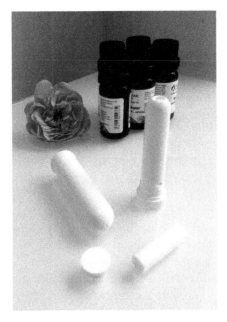

Figure 8.2. The components of an aromastick

Once an aromastick is ready for use, it needs to be correctly and helpfully labelled. Labelling should include the patient's name, the date of preparation, the initials of the aromatherapist and a blend code for the EOs. The sharing of the aromastick with another person is not recommended. In order to avoid possible substitution with inappropriate aromatic substances, the contents of the blend are not normally disclosed. If circumstances merit the production of another aromastick, this needs to be carried out with the supervision of an aromatherapist.

Essential oils

There is no need to buy any particular EO for use with HEARTS. Most organisations have their own stock of appropriate EOs and the most important thing is to find an aroma or a blend of EOs that the patient likes. From experience, some of the most popular essential oils are: bergamot (*Citrus bergamia*), frankincense (*Boswellia carterii*), lemon (*Citrus limon*), mandarin (*Citrus reticulata*), lavender (*Lavandula angustifolia*), benzoin (*Styrax benzoin*), black pepper (*Piper nigrum*), ylang-ylang (*Cananga odorata*), geranium

(*Pelargonium graveolens*) and sandalwood (*Santalum album*). Despite the expense, it may be useful to have a small amount of neroli (*Citrus aurantium*) or rose (*Rosa damascena*) for some special situations.

Using the aromastick in HEARTS

To save time, ready-made blends are prepared in advance and aromasticks are made up in batches; it can be time-consuming to make up aromasticks singly. It is also helpful to keep the blend simple – maybe using three EOs at the most. The choice of aroma can be influenced either to find a blend that is a suitable for a particular condition or an aroma that simply delights the patient.

The patient may like to take the aromastick for a 'test drive' (or a trial run) before the treatment begins. Once the patient is confident with using an aromastick s/he can use it during the treatment, or at a later time, as and when required. Written instructions must be given to the patient and some notes may also stimulate interest from visitors. A draft outline of written instructions is described in Box 8.1 (from Maycock, Mackereth and Carter 2016), and it is important that the therapist is able to demonstrate how to use the aromastick.

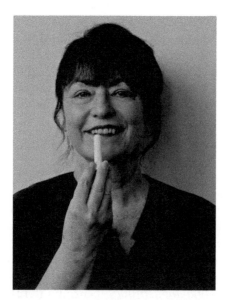

Figure 8.3. The aromastick should be held 2–3 inches (5–7 cm) from the nose

Box 8.1. How to use your aromastick

- The aromastick is for your personal use only.

- Once the outer cover has been removed, hold the stick with the perforated end towards your nose; 2–3 inches (5–7 cm) away from the nostrils is a good 'working' distance.

- Do not insert the tube into either nostril or your mouth.

- Breathe in through your nose and breathe out through your mouth using a slow, steady, comfortable breath. When you breathe in this way, the molecules of aroma have time to be adsorbed onto the sensory receptors. They will not automatically be simply blown out again. Please note that there is no special way for you to take the inbreath; it is more important that you decide what is a slow, steady breath for you.

- Repeat this comfortable pattern of breathing in and out to complete three breathing cycles. This is an easy and comfortable way to help you benefit from your aromastick.

- Repeat the breathing technique at intervals during the day, as discussed with the therapist.

- When you have finished using the aromastick, tightly replace the cover to prevent evaporation of the aroma.

- Regularly clean the inner tube surface with a clean, damp cloth or tissue.

- Never immerse the aromastick in any fluid for cleaning purposes or for any other reason.

- If you no longer need to use the aromastick, please dispose of it in general household waste. If the aroma alters, please dispose of it as above, and request a replacement if needed.

Helping patients to use an aromastick can be carried out as a demonstration and practice prior to a HEARTS treatment. Alternatively, some of the instructions that concern the breathing aspects of using the aromastick could be adapted to form a preliminary relaxation script.

Often a person will select a blend of EOs and say something like, 'That's gorgeous, it reminds me of...' This is useful information and can be linked to the patient's imagery and incorporated within the HEARTS session. Case study 8.4 describes the use of an aromastick together with some Hands-on work to help change an experience from one that was unwelcome to one that was requested.

Case study 8.4. Changing dressings – change the anchor, change the experience

Carmen was in a hospice having her medication checked. During her stay, it was necessary to change her dressing on a fungating breast ulcer on a daily basis. After day one, the nurses realised that this was not an easy task; Carmen found the procedure both distressing and painful. Medically supervised nitrous oxide inhaled gas was offered, which was helpful, but changing the dressing was still taking over half an hour. A nursing assistant (NA) suggested that some gentle stroking to Carmen's upper body and head might help, together with finding an aroma that Carmen really liked. As a result, some bergamot was put on some cotton wool and the NA started with some gentle strokes on Carmen's shoulders. She invited Carmen to pay attention to what her hands were doing as she continued with a steady rhythm and a calm voice. Carmen quickly relaxed and the dressings were changed with ease. An aromatherapist made up an aromastick for Carmen containing bergamot and frankincense that Carmen could use when the dressings were being changed. No one was surprised when Carmen asked when the dressings would be changed again!

SUMMARY

The use of aromas described in the chapter can make a valuable contribution to the HEARTS process, and can also be used in other situations. Aromas can be incorporated in a brief PCGI inspired by the patient's aroma story, facilitated by the therapist using the sensory framework. The experience and the methodology can be recalled for future self-soothing. Where EOs are available in clinical practice, aromasticks can be offered with a preferred blend identified by the patient. The chosen blend can then be incorporated within the HEARTS session and remain in the patient's possession for future use, as discussed with the therapist. Recommendations for the safe use of EOs blends have been briefly outlined within the chapter.

Part 3

HEARTS IN PRACTICE

Chapter 9

HEARTS IN CANCER CARE

KEYWORDS
cancer; co-morbidities; care pathways; HEARTS; diagnosis;
prehabilitation; treatments; fighting spirit; end of life

INTRODUCTION

This chapter presents an overview of cancer, its treatments and associated care pathways. Its purpose is to give details about the medical context in which therapists work, and to describe some of the complex issues faced by cancer patients and their families. Recommendations for good practice in clinical environments are made throughout the text of this chapter. Case studies are included to assist the reader in gaining an understanding of the benefits of offering HEARTS to patients with possible co-morbidities. Online resources that may be particularly useful are suggested in Further Reading and Online Resources at the end of the book.

THE NATURE OF CANCER AND ITS TREATMENTS

Cancer is not one disease, but a term that covers over 200 subtypes with differing prognoses, dependent on staging at diagnosis, age and gender. The aetiology is complex and there are many factors that may contribute to causality, such as genetic, viral, environmental, tobacco, alcohol and obesity factors. For a small, but significant, group of patients the cancer may be of unknown primary origin, but in recognition of this, specialist teams have emerged to optimise care in this complex area. While cancer is largely a disease of older people, it can also affect children and young adults.

For patients and families affected by cancer, everyday life can be spent dealing with symptoms, treatments and side effects that had not been planned. Patients may have other co-morbidities, such as arthritis, diabetes, dementia, heart or lung disease (NHS

England 2014). In addition to complex investigations that lead to a diagnosis, treatments can involve surgery, chemotherapy or radiotherapy, rehabilitation or palliative care. Living with cancer can create financial problems, changing relationships with family and friends, and in addition, there are the emotional sides of cancer. Comfort and contact may be impeded by the patient's condition and symptoms, such as infection, compromised immunity and isolation during radiotherapy or scanning. The person affected by cancer may perceive treatments, although potentially life-saving, as mechanistic, invasive, intrusive and associated with pain.

Over the last 20 years, the outcomes of cancer treatments have improved, with some patients being in remission and needing new care packages to manage longer-term side effects and adjusting to the 'new normal' post cancer (see Case study 9.1). However, for others, their cancers cannot be cured; the disease may progress over months or years, requiring long-term care packages, similar to other life-limiting diseases such as multiple sclerosis, diabetes and chronic obstructive pulmonary disease (COPD). There are still patients who present with cancers where the outcomes are poor, such as pancreatic and ovarian cancers, some lung cancers and brain tumours. In spite of proactive treatment, patients may progress quickly into palliative and 'end of life' care.

For improving outcomes across all cancers, prevention, early detection and rapid diagnosis is advocated, both nationally and internationally. Campaigns, such as smoking cessation, cervical screening, mammography, HPV vaccination (for females and more recently for males) and 'blood in your poo', have sought to raise public awareness and strategies for seeking help.

The range of treatment and care services is listed in Box 9.1.

Box 9.1. Treatment and care services (including innovative and novel treatments being researched and/or evaluated)

- Surgery: diagnostic, debulking and removal, stents, palliation.
- Radiotherapy techniques: linear, brachytherapy, stereotactic radiosurgery or proton beam.
- Systemic anti-cancer therapies: chemotherapy, biological/immunotherapies and/or hormone therapy.

- Palliative/symptom control interventions: steroids/non-steroidal, analgesic ladder, regional anaesthetic blocks.

- Rehabilitation: occupational therapy, physiotherapy, speech and language therapy, dietetics, survivorship programmes and living with and beyond cancer services.

- Psychological: counselling, cognitive behavioural therapy, psychotherapy and psychiatry (typically provided by specialist nurses, therapists, psychologists and psychiatrists).

- Information and support: cancer information (can also include financial, employment and benefits), complementary therapies including HEARTS, support groups/centres.

- Supportive and palliative care: family and patient support, symptom management, improving quality of life.

- End of life care: advance care planning, preferred priorities and place of care, bereavement support.

PREHABILITATION

Prehabilitation may be defined as 'Preparation around the time of cancer diagnosis, before the beginning of treatment, that includes lifestyle interventions that promote physical and psychosocial health to prepare for treatment and future impairments' (Bloom 2017). This is a process where a patient has the opportunity to learn and engage with prehabilitation strategies at diagnosis. These will continue throughout the treatment pathway, as the patient lives with and beyond cancer. The process of prehabilitation may be enhanced by introducing complementary therapies and/or HEARTS as a resource within care planning. From diagnosis throughout the cancer pathway, a therapist could become a core member of the multidisciplinary team, thus enhancing existing prehabilitation programmes and those yet to be developed.

PSYCHOLOGICAL AND SPIRITUAL CARE

In the UK, services are charged with completing a holistic needs assessment, carried out by a healthcare professional (Bloom 2017). A patient may identify his/her own needs, which could be psychological and/or spiritual, and a care plan could be developed from this process. There may be a fear of treatments and disease progression, a fear of dying, grieving over the loss of role, body image concerns, and coping with toxicities and symptoms. The origins of distress can often be multiple, such as having to deal with complex information and uncertainty, social isolation, disease progression or recurrence, and death. Coming to a 'new normal' after cancer treatment can be difficult to manage, for example, in the presence of pain and/or loss of a limb.

Coping strategies are often focused on being reactive rather than proactive. Using smoking, alcohol or recreational drugs to numb or distract from stressors can compromise health and wellbeing and undermine resilience. For some individuals, signalling severe anxiety and hopelessness will attract others who are keen to help, but these continued reactions are exhausting and can create dependency. Patients (and carers) need to be empowered to recognise care needs, and to seek information and support that promotes resilience, such as helpful self-soothing interventions and appropriate lifestyle changes. Virginia Satir (1972) has argued that it is not the problem that is the problem; rather, it is *coping* that is the problem...when patients don't have the resources to deal with a problem, they may need help to find a way of coping.

Fighting spirit activities, such as utilising support groups and making significant dietary changes, are often alluded to in the cancer literature (Lepore *et al.* 2014; Wilkinson *et al.* 2012). If these changes are not maintained, there can be feelings of guilt and failure, especially if the disease progresses or recurs (Watson *et al.* 1999). It is important to state that however well equipped a patient is to deal with cancer, there are always times when it will all be too much. A HEARTS experience can offer a patient an opportunity for becoming calm, even feeling content in the moment, and holding the memory for future recall (see Case study 9.2). HEARTS can also contribute to self-care through the patient recalling the HEARTS experience and enabling carers to deliver an intervention when a therapist is not able to be present.

For some patients, 'end of life' may be the next stage. This can create an existential crisis that can be an opportunity for planning and making peace with one's self and with others (Mackereth and Dunn 2017). A cancer diagnosis and all that it entails can be challenging and distressing for carers as they witness a loved one going through investigations, treatments and disease processes and symptoms (see Case study 9.5). HEARTS has a potential role to play through promoting calm and sleep, offering comfort and helping to create positive memories that can become a resource for the future.

TO WHOM AND WHEN TO OFFER HEARTS

HEARTS can help relieve some of the distress and emotional symptoms of the cancer journey. Numerous case studies, the results from the questionnaire (see Chapter 12) and experience have suggested that HEARTS is suitable for patients, carers and staff affected by cancer at any point on the pathway. Sometimes therapists regard HEARTS as a therapeutic approach that is only for use in palliative care and at end of life, or when a complementary therapy is not considered to be suitable for the patient. Deciding not to offer HEARTS may not be in the patient's best interests. Some patients have reservations about 'touchy feely' interventions and acquiesce to the support, only to be surprised by their own responses to the intervention. The patient's competence to consent must be assured and advice can be sought from the patient's named nurse or key worker.

PREPARATION AND SAFETY ISSUES IN CLINICAL ENVIRONMENTS

1. Assessing the environment

Most therapists will want to become involved with treating the patient as soon as they possibly can to make the most of the time available. In the questionnaire results (see Chapter 12), eight respondents questioned the suitability of the treatment space and the need to negotiate around clinical equipment as both a concern and a constraint. We suggest that before becoming involved, the therapist makes an assessment of the environment and considers his/her approach with the minimum of disturbance for the patient.

On the macro level, noise may be integral, and it is not possible to make changes, for example, the noise of an infusion pump, telephones ringing and ongoing conversations that can sometimes be intrusive. It may not be possible to completely screen an area for a patient and this may not be desirable – the patient may not want the curtains drawn around his/her bed. When arranging the bed and the pillows be considerate of oxygen masks, intravenous cannulas and tubing from catheters and drains, so the patient also realises you are taking care with his/her clinical treatments.

2. Hygiene and infection control

On the micro level, choosing a texture with which to cover the patient may be limited to the hospital or hospice linen. For many patients, skin integrity and risk of bruising due to a low platelet count requires therapists to inform patients (and colleagues) that the touch technique is light and unlikely to cause any tissue damage or bruising. Infection control can present challenges for the use of massage where the skin is disturbed. However, even when the therapist is working over a fabric of some kind, for example, a towel, sheet, bedcover or dressing gown, it is important to adhere to infection control procedures, for example, the therapist's arms should be bare below the elbows. Hygiene policies, including hand drying and the appropriate use of alcohol hand rubs, must also be adhered to.

3. The therapist's posture and access to the patient

A patient's position can also present challenges, not only for the patient's personal comfort, but also for the person delivering HEARTS. For example, a breathless patient may wish to remain fully upright, sitting in a chair, or s/he may be lying on his/her side. The therapist needs to decide how best to work with what s/he finds, rather than expecting a patient to move, or to try to assist the patient in moving. Sometimes in challenging situations a second therapist may be able to assist, so that one therapist works on one area of the patient while the other therapist works on a different area. Two therapists working together may offer easier access to the patient (see Chapter 6).

It is helpful to check out with the patient whether a position is comfortable by making a closed question, 'Is this better or worse?' This provides a limited choice of response, and the therapist is more likely to get a focused answer, such as, 'No, it was better where it was.' If the patient is asked an open question, such as, 'How is that for you?', the answer is more likely to be, 'That's fine', as some patients may not want to disappoint the therapist by being truthful (see Chapter 5).

4. The patient's wishes relating to the presence of carers or staff

The patient needs to agree to the presence of staff and/or carers in the immediate area of his/her bed or chair. Sometimes observers or visitors feel they should comment, and it may be helpful if the therapist suggests that the observers or visitors may like to 'get comfortable' in a chair and listen to the therapist's voice as the intervention continues (see Chapter 11 for 'bystander effects'). As part of learning to practise HEARTS, carers (or staff) may want to contribute to the intervention, but once again, their level of participation must be agreed beforehand with the patient.

5. Agreeing boundaries

It helps to create trust if the patient has the opportunity to say if there is any area where s/he does not want to receive touch. This is also essential to the consent process at the start of treatment. Consent needs to be ongoing – at any point the patient may want to stop or take a break. A simple hand gesture that has been agreed will suffice (for example, the hand signal with the raised palm that signals 'STOP'), and must be respected.

6. Communicating with the patient about concerns

It may be useful, but not necessary, to ask how the patient (or carer) feels at the beginning of the treatment. However, asking about a specific concern could bring attention to it, so mentioning a symptom, such as pain or nausea, may be counterproductive. It is better to be 'artfully vague', by staying in the present as you work with HEARTS. If the patient mentions a symptom(s), the therapist could say something like, 'Whatever issue or concern is of importance to you, just make a note, and then listen to my voice helping you to create a sense of calm, which is travelling through your arms and into your hands...' The therapist can ask for feedback at intervals during the treatment, although it is not necessary to do this continuously. A simple gesture or a nod or a smile from the patient will serve as a response, or even stating that you will make a note of it and discuss it further at the end of the session.

7. Acknowledging vulnerable/sensitive areas of the body

As the intervention proceeds, it is important to acknowledge any equipment in place or area of compromised skin integrity, such as a cannula or drain, or bruising or inflammation – for example, 'I am carefully working above your arm/hand with the intravenous cannula in place.' For someone with oxygen therapy or where a nebuliser is running, you could even suggest, 'The oxygen might have a helpful colour that can flow to a part that needs oxygenation and a feeling of calm.'

8. Maintaining records of an intervention

A key part of the process is to record or document the intervention according to the care setting policy, importantly using the patient's words in terms of feedback in the record. Additionally, recording consent, the date and time spent with the patient and signing the entry is essential to any documentation if a paper record. Some care settings will hold electronic records and the therapist will need to have completed the appropriate training and adherence to clinical governance and confidentiality policies.

EXAMPLES OF HEARTS CASE STUDIES IN ACUTE CARE

Case study 9.1. Feeling normal again

Earlier in the chapter, learning to live with a 'new normal' was mentioned. The patient in this case study was attempting to adjust to living with constant pain following a leg amputation.

In offering HEARTS to Amir six weeks after a right hindquarter amputation for osteosarcoma, Amir said that he was experiencing constant pain in the now phantom leg. The hip pain was due to a sense that the leg was being twisted outwards and away from him. The pain radiated from the top of his leg to his toes. The HEARTS sequence involved gentle holding over the hips and legs (imagining the missing limb present) combined with breathing techniques, guided imagery and breeze strokes above the missing leg. At the end of this session, Amir said the twisty sensation remained but the pain had gone in both the hip and leg.

A second treatment was offered a week later. The gentle holding was repeated with more focus on a sense of release within the hip area. At the end of the session Amir felt that his phantom leg was straight. He described the sensation as 'feeling normal' again. He was very excited to tell his surgeon about HEARTS and the perceived outcome.

Case study 9.2. Being smoke-free with HEARTS

A diagnosis of cancer can trigger a major change of lifestyle. Maurice, who was in his 60s, had lung cancer, COPD and diabetes. He had been admitted to hospital for stabilising his diabetes and other symptoms. On many occasions he had heard that stopping smoking could help with his peripheral neuropathy and breathlessness. The smoking cessation advisor (SCA) had offered nicotine replacement therapy, but Maurice refused. The SCA suggested seeing a complementary therapist so he could use his time in hospital (which was a smoke-free zone) to go 'cold turkey' supported by some relaxation therapy. Maurice rejected reflexology because of problems with peripheral neuropathy, but was intrigued by her description of HEARTS. A therapist visited Maurice, and after a 20-minute session that focused on Maurice's arms, shoulders, head and face, he whispered quietly, 'I am content. You can go now.' The therapist suggested that Maurice could use the memory of the session to recall the 'content' as a means of going smoke-free and helping his symptoms. Maurice liked this approach and felt it would help his journey to becoming smoke-free, and requested further sessions.

Case study 9.3. HEARTS after major surgery

Pain and discomfort can become so intrusive it can be overwhelming and debilitating. In this case study a surgical patient was helped to begin her recovery through the use of HEARTS.

The therapist was asked to see a young woman, Sandy, who had received major breast surgery two days previously. The patient's left arm was painful around the shoulder joint and she believed that her arm had been in an awkward position for a considerable amount of time during the operation.

Not knowing quite what to do, the therapist used gentle stroking movements along Sandy's body, together with therapeutic holding. She noticed how quickly the patient relaxed, and after gaining the patient's permission, the therapist moved to the shoulder that was painful and began therapeutic holding. After a few minutes, she felt that it might be helpful to hold the patient's arm and support it so that the therapist was taking all the weight of the arm. Gradually the arm became heavier and heavier, and when the therapist felt it was too heavy to hold any longer, she gently placed the arm on the bed and concluded the treatment. That afternoon, a request came from the ward for 'some more of what the therapist did this morning'. So next morning, the therapist did a repeat of the HEARTS treatment she had done on the previous day. The patient was delighted, and reported how the pain had eased and how much better she felt. A third appointment was made for the following day, but in the meantime, Sandy was discharged. She was upset that she wouldn't be able to access HEARTS outside the hospital environment.

Case study 9.4. HEARTS at the end of life

Sleep disturbances are not uncommon at any point during treatment and beyond. At end of life there can be a fear of sleeping because the patient may be fearful that s/he may die while asleep. This case study describes how HEARTS helped a young man to sleep at the end of life.

Tom was a young man in his early 20s who was entering the end of life with a progressive disease. Although his preferred place for care was home, his complex needs had resulted in a hospice admission for symptom management. He found this new environment 'a bit posh' and was having trouble sleeping. Two nursing assistants (NAs) with HEARTS training offered Tom a session with relaxing music playing softly in the background. They decided to deliver a HEARTS sequence that involved stroking his arms from his shoulder to his hands, using the same speed, the same rhythm and matching the pressure they were using as much as they could. After a few minutes, Tom's eyes closed and the NAs continued with the rhythmic stroking until his breathing changed and they saw he was asleep. Three hours later, when Tom awoke, he said, 'Whatever did you two do to me? I have never had sleep like that in my whole life.' The two NAs continued to carry out short HEARTS treatments for Tom every few days. Interestingly, although Tom did wake during the night, he did not require any further sleep medication until he died a few weeks later.

Case study 9.5. HEARTS and rallying at the end of life

Bhavan, in his 60s, had advanced metastatic disease from a bowel primary, although the reason for admitting him to the hospice was for pneumonia. The medical team had prescribed antibiotics and hydration, but had advised his partner Bibi that end of life was highly likely. Bibi was not accepting of this prognosis, and appeared distressed.

The nurse asked the HEARTS therapist to visit Bibi and Bhavan to see if there was anything she could do to help. Bibi took the opportunity to go for a walk, leaving the therapist gently holding Bhavan's feet. The therapist did not feel this was enough, so she continued with therapeutic holding of the 'landmarks' (see Chapter 6), and speaking quietly to him as she did so. As the therapist worked, she noticed Bhavan's breathing noticeably seemed more comfortable, and his whole body looked more relaxed. Bibi returned and noticed the changes and called the nurse. On examination, the nurse said his vital signs appeared stronger. Bhavan rallied over the next few days and was discharged home. The therapist taught Bibi the sequence she had used, adding some of the stroking movements. This practice became part of Bibi and Bhavan's daily routine until two months later, when Bhavan died peacefully at home.

Case study 9.6. HEARTS, post treatment and intimate relationships

The following community-based case study illustrates the potential of HEARTS on sexual wellbeing.

Jim had prostate cancer with metastatic disease. He was devoted to his partner, but on the first visit to the therapist, he tentatively disclosed that their sex life was not what it once was. He felt that he had let her down and he was feeling very stressed as he didn't know how to cope with this new situation. The therapist suggested that he might like to experience a HEARTS session in the first instance. At the end of the 25-minute treatment, Jim said, 'I feel quite different – more like the old Jim.' He was grateful that someone with whom he did not have an intimate relationship could touch him in such a caring way. The therapist suggested that this was something he could share with his partner. At the next visit, he said that just stroking and holding each other, and cuddling up on the settee had been wonderful in helping them to relax. They felt much closer to each other and the therapist's suggestion had made them both very happy.

SUMMARY

This chapter has outlined the nature of cancer and the current treatment and care pathways. Good practice has been advocated in the section on preparation and safety issues in clinical environments. The anonymised case studies in this chapter demonstrate the use of HEARTS with patients affected by cancer at different stages of the cancer journey. Cancer is so diverse and we had many more case histories than we could include, so we selected some of the main ones. They were grouped together to try and give the reader the diversity of situations in which HEARTS could be used. The heading of each case history should be a sufficient descriptor of the nature of each situation.

Chapter 10

DEMENTIA AND MEMORY LOSS

KEYWORDS
HEARTS; dementia; memory loss;
touch hunger; carer involvement; consent

INTRODUCTION

This chapter explores the role of HEARTS for older people living with cancer. Aside from cancers being a common occurrence as we age, there may be the added complications of already living with other co-morbidities, including memory loss or dementia. A relative or partner living with someone with cancer may have dementia or memory loss, often leading to difficult situations and complex challenges with the patient's care and treatment. For example, it is possible that a familial carer witnessing a loved one undergoing cancer investigations and treatments may become overwhelmed and distressed. HEARTS can provide therapeutic opportunities to utilise touch in assisting with communication, providing comfort and an experience of being cared for, all of which can ease distress and promote resilience. To explore the application of HEARTS in this context, issues related to consent, and working with familial carers and supporting staff, are addressed through utilising case studies and identifying recommendations for best practice. Please note that the term 'caregiver' in this chapter can include a relative or friend, or a member of staff in a care or nursing home.

SOME CHALLENGES OF GROWING OLDER

The Hollywood actress Bette Davis is said to have stated that, 'growing old isn't for sissies'. We all need to be careful when making assumptions about what ageing means for an individual. For some, it can be a time to be free from work routines and the responsibilities of childcare, to focus on themselves, their interests and new adventures. Some older people can feel liberated and less inhibited as their choices and lifestyle changes may surprise and even raise concern among family and friends. Many older relatives cherish time spent with grandchildren, nieces and nephews, but usually, at the end of the day, these 'charges' are then handed back to their parents. While ageing does not always correlate with disease and disability, the impact of these can be an everyday reality for many older people. Conditions such as diabetes, arthritis, heart and lung diseases often require ongoing medical care that may limit activities and independence. Advances in drug and other therapies have reduced the illness burden for many, but these may also come with side effects and the need for monitoring. As we grow older with one or more health concerns, fear and anxiety may inhibit how we engage socially, and with activities that require effort, mobility and flexibility.

Smoking and alcohol use increase the risk for many cancers, including lung, head and neck cancers, and these behaviours are also linked to a greater risk of dementia (García, Ramón-Bou and Porta 2010; Syrigos *et al.* 2009). Memory loss and differing forms of dementia present patients and their caregivers with challenges on a cancer journey. For example, possible symptoms of cancer may be ignored or not reported by the patient or carer. This can contribute to a late diagnosis being made, with an increased risk of poor outcomes for people affected by memory loss and/or dementia (Solomons, Solomons and Gosney 2013).

According to the National Institute on Aging (NIA), 'dementia' is an umbrella term for a set of symptoms including impaired thinking, memory loss, language and problem-solving difficulties. Dementia is caused when the brain is damaged by disease, such as Alzheimer's disease, the presence of Lewy bodies or vascular disease. Dementia is generally progressive, which means the symptoms will get worse. This deterioration can be accelerated with further stresses and disease burden. Another layer of complication is the differential diagnosis of confusion, delirium, depression and cognitive and behavioural changes. Additionally, these complications may be triggered by infection, dehydration and even some medications, such as steroids and sedation (Polson and Croy 2015).

Dementia care nurse specialists, dementia care training courses and initiatives such as 'Dementia Friends' seek to share knowledge, reduce the stigma of dementia and improve care in a range of clinical and care settings. It is also important to assess the environment of care, the availability of memory boxes containing familiar items, such as pictures of loved ones, and access to music and activities that engage and bring comfort (Handley, Bunn and Goodman 2017).

TOUCH HUNGER, CANCER CARE AND OLDER PEOPLE

Older people are particularly vulnerable to 'touch hunger', a need for tactile communication and comfort, which, if provided, could decrease a sense of isolation and loneliness (see Chapter 2). It may be that partners and friends have died, family members may have moved away, or it may only be possible to see elderly relatives rarely. Montagu (1986, p.34) states that '...tactile needs do not seem to change with ageing...if anything, the need tends to increase'. It could be argued that while grandchildren are infants, society expects grandparents to play a major role in a grandchild's life. Grandchildren like to sit on granny or grandpa's lap, listen to stories and interact playfully, often with hugs and kisses. However, as the grandchildren grow up, their peer groups become more important, and physical contact with the grandparents usually diminishes (see Chapter 2). Unfortunately, we also live in a society where many people are increasingly wary of touch and being tactile with others, particularly as touching may be misinterpreted as having a sexual/ abusive intent (Field 2014).

Institutions can develop a clinical culture that becomes so hampered by risk-averse professional boundaries that compassionate touch is feared and then becomes lost as a caring norm. For the patient who is both distressed and fearful of cancer, which may be perceived as a terminal illness, there is a searching for a hand to hold. Touch hunger may be familiar to therapists and caregivers who work with older people in care settings. We are all familiar with the situation where an older person takes hold of an offered hand, which s/he grips firmly and is reluctant to release. Knowing how to respond to touch hunger within a prescribed role can raise conflicts for professional caregivers. They may struggle with offering compassionate touch, fearful that it could be time-consuming and overwhelming, particularly when there are competing role demands. HEARTS could offer a short intervention that offers meaningful contact with a sense of purpose and a boundary, and once learned, is within the skill set of most caregivers, including family members.

For a patient and his/her carers, a double diagnosis of cancer and dementia can be very frightening. The number of individuals having both conditions is increasing, partly related to individuals living to an older age. It is also possible that an older couple might include one person with cancer and another with dementia. Until a diagnosis of cancer, the partner or the patient who is living with early dementia (and/or significant memory loss) may have coped at home. However, when a carer is confronted with caring for someone with cancer, s/he can become easily stressed, overwhelmed and then risk further deterioration. In our experience, it is not unusual for HEARTS to be a powerful experience for a distressed carer who is witnessing a calming and rhythmic intervention for a loved one (see Case study 10.1). This phenomenon has been described as the 'bystander effect', which is possibly a form of 'somatic resonance' (Ross 2000) linked to an empathetic response. Being close to a recipient of HEARTS, both emotionally and physically, triggers a shared sense of calm, time distortion and possibly a relaxation response (see also Chapters 11 and 12).

Case study 10.1. A shared wait for morphine and release with HEARTS

Jill was a caregiver in a nursing home. One evening she was checking on the residents for whom she cared when she found Eileen sitting by her mother, Mary, who had early stage dementia. Eileen turned to Jill and said, 'Isn't there anything that you can do?' Jill had only recently completed the HEARTS introductory training, but thought that HEARTS might help. First, Jill asked Mary if it was okay to place her hands gently on Mary's ankles and to do some gentle stroking movements on her lower legs. Mary nodded, and at first there seemed to be little response. Jill then decided to include her voice and commented on the slow rhythmic stroking movements as she delivered them. After five minutes of watching Jill work, Mary closed her eyes and fell asleep for over three hours. It was only when Jill had finished the short treatment that Eileen took her aside and said, 'Thank you so much. My mum has been diagnosed with cancer and we were waiting for the morphine, which is why I think she was so agitated. Please can you show me what I can do, so I can help my mother when you are not around?' She added, 'You know, just watching you treating my mum made me feel so calm, I lost track of time, it was as if you were also comforting me at the same time. I couldn't stop yawning and felt like taking a nap next to my mum.'

CHALLENGES FOR CARERS

For caregivers, whether family or in a professional capacity, dementia presents an additional burden through the cancer journey, with numerous challenging behaviours and uncertainty as to how to respond compassionately. For example, 'sundowning' is a symptom of Alzheimer's disease and other forms of dementia (also known as 'late-day confusion'; Canevelli *et al.* 2016). The patient's confusion and agitation may worsen during the late afternoon and evening, although these symptoms may be less pronounced earlier in the day. Confusion may also be linked to early stage dementia, which may be exacerbated by an underlying infection, constipation, medication or dehydration. Fear and distress may be associated with earlier experiences, for example, trauma, sexual abuse or wartime imprisonment. In a pilot randomised controlled study, Suzuki *et al.* (2010) found that sessions of tactile touch appeared to assist in reducing agitation and aggression; both symptoms can be difficult symptoms to manage.

The challenges of investigations and cancer treatments are that patients need to understand what is happening and be able to follow instructions, for example, lying still during a physical examination or the placement of an intravenous cannula. Patients may be required to attend daily for short treatments of radiotherapy, which may include the use of a protective and stabilising mould or mask to protect areas of the body not affected by cancer. It is possible to elicit consent in the moment; the challenge is to maintain the consent throughout a procedure. With the creative use of touch, the voice and the pace at which you speak, the components of HEARTS can be utilised to promote comfort and calm, even in complex situations (see Case study 10.2 and also Chapter 7).

When working with someone affected by dementia and cancer we need to have a consistent pattern of intervention and continuity of support for each session. The therapeutic work described in the case study below was facilitated by two therapists who were able to maintain a relationship with the patient, the carer and radiotherapy staff (Hackman *et al.* 2013).

Case study 10.2. Agitation, in the moment consent and singing 'Yellow Submarine'

Don, aged 67, had been living with dementia since his mid-50s. He had a history of smoking and alcohol use, and had recently been diagnosed with oral cancer. The tumour had been removed and he was due for 20 sessions of daily radiotherapy. He appeared to understand his diagnosis, but after 10 minutes of wearing the mask during radiotherapy, he would forget where he was and become agitated. On the second session, therapists were asked to provide an intervention to help him settle during mask placement and treatment. Don was asked about his favourite piece of music and place. He talked about his daughter, during a time when she was poorly. Don remembered singing 'Yellow Submarine' by the Beatles, and gently stroking her arms and legs, which had helped her during a hospital stay. For the next treatment, two therapists accompanied Don. One organised the music and sang along to it, while the other therapist gently held and stroked Don's arms and legs while repeating back the story that Don had shared. During the radiotherapy, the therapist continued to talk to Don over the intercom, with the second therapist interspersing the story of the 'Yellow Submarine' and singing the chorus. He was able to successfully complete 17 of the radiotherapy sessions, and the medical team decided that was sufficient. Don recovered well from radiotherapy and continued to be supported at home by an Admiral nurse/dementia nurse specialist.

MAKING THE MOST OF TEXTURES AND FAMILIAR ITEMS

Textures can have a major role to play a part in a HEARTS intervention; these may include a familiar blanket, a treasured scarf or shawl or even a 'twiddle muff' (see Figure 10.1).

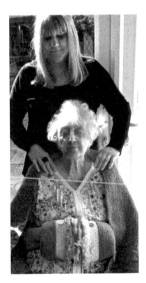

Figure 10.1. Working with HEARTS, using a home-knitted blanket and a twiddle muff that contained buttons on the inside

Sensory experience of familiar materials and items can evoke kinaesthetic memories by engaging the patient 'in the moment', together with their own sensory comfort (see Chapter 2). The caregiver can incorporate the characteristics of a blanket within the HEARTS intervention. S/he can bring attention to the history of the item, and invite the person to, 'become aware of the colours, the textures, the weight and the warmth, noticing how comfy it feels'. It is important to acknowledge that the positive intention behind incorporating a blanket is as important than the words. It may also help to ask family members about the significance and history of the blanket (or a scarf or shawl) to ensure that it is appropriate and could hold helpful memories.

Attention can be drawn to the covering at various stages of the delivery of HEARTS, and the caregiver's stories can be woven in and out of the Hands-on work, finally ensuring the blanket is available for the next session (see Case study 10.3).

Sensory experience of familiar materials and items can evoke kinaesthetic memories by engaging the person in the moment and may contribute to his/her sense of sensory comfort (see Chapter 2). Items that may be useful for the patient to hold may be a treasured watch, an item of jewellery, a souvenir from a special event – or anything that has positive meaning for the patient.

Case study 10.3. The comforting memories of textures – an experience worthy of repeat

Mike, aged 78, with prostate cancer and dementia, was being cared for within a residential home. As his disease progressed he had episodes of shouting and repeating of words, so much so that carers struggled to calm him, particularly at night. With permission from his partner, Joan, two caregivers offered to provide HEARTS, incorporating a homemade blanket that Mike was attached to. Placing the blanket lightly over his chest and arms, the caregivers talked to Mike about the coloured squares and textures of the yarn while stroking downwards from his shoulders to his fingers, incorporating stillness by stopping and holding at frequent intervals. Mike reached for one of the caregiver's hands and gave it a squeeze and smiled. She smiled back and said, 'Can I continue to gently stroke your arms and hands over this lovely blanket that Joan made?' One of the caregivers asked if they could continue stroking down the outside of his Mike's legs. He had stopped shouting and was calm enough to nod. Gradually, Mike closed his eyes and drifted off to sleep. The caregivers incorporated the routine each evening, which seemed to help with reducing the number of 'shouting' episodes at night. Mike died a month later; Joan took the blanket home to place on their bed.

CREATING A LASTING MEMORY

Teaching familial carers can be very helpful, particularly if they can provide the intervention once the patient has been discharged from a hospital for hospice (see Chapter 11). For those patients and families at end of life, there is an opportunity to provide a shared experience. In bereavement, this can assist with the family's wellbeing, informing their memories from a caring experience. Sometimes families will not always be able to acknowledge the value of a moment until it becomes a memory (Duhamel 1919) (see Case study 10.4).

Case study 10.4. HEARTS for both the carer and patient

Martha, aged 60, had early stage dementia and lung cancer and had been admitted to a hospice from home to improve her breathlessness and a cough. A nursing assistant and a member of the care home team used the Library of Strokes from HEARTS when Martha was distressed and agitated. Fortunately, both had learned HEARTS and used light, rhythmic finger stroking and gentle holding of Martha's knees and legs. They talked to her in a relaxed tone, and showed empathy and respect while they used fingertip brushing. This therapeutic intervention had a beneficial effect on Martha who became calmer and less agitated. The benefit of the treatment was acknowledged by medical staff who could see a difference in Martha's distress and agitation. Martha's partner, Ingrid, asked the caregivers if they would teach her so she could provide HEARTS at home. The caregiver said 'Yes' and added, 'How would it be if we treat both of you at the same time, then you would have a memory of receiving HEARTS to inform your learning?' Ingrid acknowledged she was tired and that, 'It would be a lovely thing to have.' The reclining chair in the room was used, with pillows to support her arms, which mirrored Martha's position on a treatment couch. The caregivers started at the same time using towels as a cover, with one caregiver leading the Library of Strokes as the other repeated the movements with Ingrid. At the end of the session both Martha and Ingrid had drifted into relaxation, well supported by the pillows. Ingrid emerged from a 10-minute doze and hugged the caregiver.

USING THE AROMA MEMORY

The smell memory of familiar everyday substances can play a useful role in HEARTS and dementia and cancer care. Although the patient may not be able to recall the verbal name of the smell, it is likely that a family member would know what it is. It may be something like a favourite perfume, aftershave, a brand of soap, polish, home cleaners – the list of possibilities is endless. A family member could bring in the source of the aroma so it could be present in the room. Alternatively, the therapist could invite a memory of the aroma to be recalled during the HEARTS intervention (see Chapter 8). A family member could be asked to help construct the imagery, and then it could be relayed back to the patient in a story form that could include the names of family members who had an association with the aroma. Reactions to aromas can change; it is important to acknowledge that disease, medication and injury may affect the olfactory receptor sites and neurological pathways. It is also important to acknowledge that memories of aromas can linger from early childhood, informing reactions, both positively and negatively, to current contact with aromas (Herz 2009; Levy *et al.* 1999). Aromasticks may also have a useful role to play. It may be that if the patient is cognitively able to engage with choosing an aromastick from a small selection, this can be used along with the Hands-on work, as described in Chapter 5.

RECOMMENDATIONS

- HEARTS can be easily learned by caregivers in residential homes/elderly care settings and can be a useful adjunct to activities of daily living such as washing, getting dressed, after combing hair or before bed time.

- When working with an individual who has memory loss or dementia, gather information and advice from the nursing staff/caregivers as to how dementia is affecting the patient.

- Seek guidance and information about the patient's ability to consent in the moment and for how long s/he can maintain this consent.

- If the patient is unable to give verbal or written consent, identify non-verbal cues that can be elicited and monitored, to ensure that the patient is maintaining consent.

- Involve a family carer when possible, for example, by enabling the carer to be present or ideally assisting with HEARTS delivery.

- Find out which approaches might be most helpful – perhaps try out two to three methods from the Library of Strokes or palming.

- Do not try and do too much in one session. Note verbal and non-verbal cues that indicate enjoyment and comfort, or cues that signal the need to stop and review.

- Maintain communication and contact. Do not challenge or correct the patient when s/he talks about the date, events or memories that are shared as though they are in the present rather than in the past.

- Remember that a patient may find it hard to maintain contact if s/he cannot see or hear you. It is important to remember this as you position yourself relative to the patient.

- Repeat who you are and the name of the person assisting with HEARTS, whenever introducing the next stage of the intervention; this may be a familiar caregiver. The patient might become anxious searching his/her memory for your name and what you are doing, etc.

- Maintain a calm, open manner, using words that are soothing, calming and inviting.

- When an individual is anxious, his/her mouth can become dry, so it's harder to speak and clear the throat. Offering water periodically can be useful to ensure hydration and comfort.

- Be aware that the intervention may be interrupted by the need to go to the toilet or for the person to talk or reminisce. HEARTS may also act as a trigger to positive memories. Sharing a lovely memory may bring comfort in the moment, even if the individual forgets who you are or what is happening today, for example, a medical treatment or investigation.

SUMMARY

When dementia is present alongside cancer, the co-morbidity of the two illnesses can add another level of complexity to care, so there is a need to adapt interventions to best fit the situation encountered. This chapter has covered the challenges faced by patients and carers who find themselves in this situation, and the role that HEARTS can play in patient care has been discussed. Case histories have been included to demonstrate how HEARTS can be integrated into patient care. Recommendations have been made in terms of how the therapist relates to the patient. Where dementia is present, HEARTS can offer an engaging package of care with its inclusivity of touch, a 'comfy' textile, meaningful imagery and aromas.

Chapter 11

LEARNING AND TEACHING HEARTS

Keywords
teaching; HEARTS; microteaching; motivation; learning styles;
therapists; healthcare professionals; carers; bystander effect

INTRODUCTION

This chapter focuses on the learning and teaching of the HEARTS Process for therapists and carers. The first section overviews training for complementary therapists who specialise in cancer care, and healthcare professionals who are interested in the skilful use of touch in the course of their work. It includes a description of current courses and makes recommendations for further developments. The second section begins with a brief exploration of the challenges of being a carer. This is followed by a description of the approaches that therapists can use to assist carers in learning the principles of HEARTS. Some of the results from Question 11 in the questionnaire are referred to in this chapter, as the responses support the purposeful use of HEARTS for carers (see also Chapter 12).

SECTION 1. A BRIEF HISTORY OF HEARTS TRAINING

HEARTS training began around 1995 as one- or two-day courses entitled 'Touch Therapy'. Initially, the two-day courses were held on single days that were a fortnight apart – the intention was to give participants the opportunity to practise between the two days. However, participants couldn't always attend the second day, the travelling costs of attending two days increased, and not everyone was able to practise between the two days. Additionally, and as the content of HEARTS developed, it became more acceptable for participants to attend the training on two consecutive days. However, a two-day course was not appropriate for some professional settings, so the content was modified to enable a one-day 'introductory' workshop to be delivered for some target groups, for example, care home staff, community nurses and nursing assistants. The content has been refined to safely equip carers (often working in care and nursing homes) to deliver a short HEARTS intervention as part of their caring roles.

The two-day course is designed for complementary therapists and healthcare professionals who have either a complementary therapy qualification or an interest in integrating skilful touch in their professional roles. On occasions, healthcare professionals have been motivated to take up complementary therapy training. One student described the HEARTS introductory workshop as a turning point in her career path. She left her job and focused on complementary therapies. Her current career is in providing a range of therapies, including HEARTS, for people living with cancer.

Currently, over 1000 therapists and healthcare professionals have been formally trained to deliver HEARTS to patients and carers in the UK, Ireland and Canada. Their backgrounds are from a range of healthcare settings, for example, acute cancer care, hospice, home care and support facilities for people with longer-term conditions such as Down's syndrome, multiple sclerosis, Parkinson's disease and dementia care.

More recently, 15 experienced HEARTS practitioners have completed the HEARTS teacher training course at the Integrative Therapies Training Unit at The Christie.[1] These teachers are now delivering one- and two-day courses across the UK and Ireland. With the publication of this book, together with more planned training courses, the provision of HEARTS within healthcare settings is set to increase. See Box 11.1 for a summary of the three approaches to HEARTS training.

---

1   The Christie NHS Trust is a major cancer hospital in Manchester, in the North West of England.

Box 11.1. HEARTS training

1. The introductory HEARTS course

This group includes mainly non-complementary therapists and those who have healthcare training. Carers from nursing homes and care homes have also benefited from this training and have been able to extend the amount and quality of touch they use when caring for residents. Course participants receive training to deliver safely a modified 5- to 15-minute HEARTS intervention. The content focuses on an explanation of HEARTS, the potential role of touch in everyday care, the strokedown and the use of the voice and obtaining consent. Sometimes guidance is introduced by the organisation to enable participants to carry out the practice of HEARTS. Depending on the needs of the organisation, this one-day course can also be held for other groups such as hospice nurses and nursing assistants.

2. The therapists' HEARTS training course

This practical course is designed for qualified, experienced and insured complementary therapists, and includes all the aspects of HEARTS. The aim is to equip complementary therapists to integrate and safely adapt HEARTS interventions for patients and carers within a range of healthcare settings.

In addition to the material in the one-day course, there is development of the Library of Strokes, the use of the voice and aromas, together with issues of consent and introducing HEARTS into the workplace.

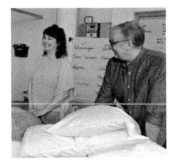

*Participants tell us that all our HEARTS courses
are relaxing and fun, and they take away new
techniques to use with patients and carers*

Within six months of completing the course, students have the option of submitting two case studies to be considered for being awarded the HEARTS practitioner certificate as recognition of their practice. Feedback about the content of their case histories is given to the student in writing by the course tutor.

3. Teaching the HEARTS Process

This course is a recent addition, and is currently being run at the Christie Integrative Therapies Training Unit. It is only open to therapists who have completed the two-day HEARTS training course and who have some experience of working with HEARTS in patient care. The content includes the principles and practice of teaching HEARTS and evaluating future training courses. The course is limited to eight participants, as the content includes a supported microteaching session, with all students delivering an adapted HEARTS training session for 20 minutes plus 10 minutes of feedback. Support and mentoring are offered to the trainees on an ongoing basis after the course is completed.

RECOMMENDATIONS FOR FUTURE HEARTS TEACHERS' COURSES

As the teacher training course is a relatively new addition to the HEARTS training programme, it has not yet been possible to introduce firm criteria for training standards. To date, all the participants have been known to the course facilitator, and are known to be experienced therapists working in supportive and palliative care settings. Some participants have assisted on previous HEARTS two-day courses where these have been available. Ideally, criteria for admission to the teacher training courses need to be developed along with ongoing mentoring for HEARTS teachers; these are two aspects of the HEARTS teachers' course that are currently being explored.

SECTION 2. CARERS AND HEARTS

It could be argued that the quickest way to reinforce skills is to teach another person in the real world of care. From our survey, which is reported in detail in Chapter 12, carers were reported as being impressed with the outcomes of HEARTS, and many were curious and eager to learn themselves. For some, this was so they could deliver an intervention either at home, or during visiting, when a therapist or health professional might not be available. In this section, case studies and responses from our survey are included to illustrate the theory and practice of teaching carers.

SOME CHALLENGES OF BEING A CARER

Cancer and other life-limiting diseases affect both the patient and the lives of families and friends (see Chapter 9). Campbell and Knowles (2016) acknowledge that carers, as well as patients, are experiencing high levels of stress. In addition to supporting their loved one, carers put their own lives on hold and may need to juggle family life and their jobs together with the shock and implications of a diagnosis of cancer or another life-limiting illness. Carers may find themselves keeping a 'vigil at the bedside' and although fatigued, and at times overwhelmed, many are reluctant to either request some complementary therapy for themselves or to accept it when it is offered (Mackereth *et al.* 2014). Sometimes, the carer may refuse; s/he may believe that patients are the priority, they have the most need, and it is the patient who should receive whatever supportive care is available. However, the patient does not always share this view; often s/he will want the carer to have something for him or herself. It is likely that the patient may feel better and more relaxed when s/he is aware that the carer is receiving something of benefit.

WITNESSING HEARTS: IMPRESSED AND 'PLEASE CAN I LEARN?'

In the HEARTS questionnaire (see Chapter 12), therapists (*n*=38) were asked to report any unsolicited comments received from carers/ family members who were present during a HEARTS treatment for their loved one. Carers observing HEARTS treatments readily identified the benefits of HEARTS treatments for patients. One respondent commented: *He has fallen asleep... I have never seen him so relaxed since his diagnosis* (R4F) and a second observed ...*it [HEARTS] really calms her...you take such good care of her* (R1F). (Codes used: respondent (R), with a respondent number and stated gender, for example, R2M (male) or R3F (female).)

Two respondents implied that the effects of HEARTS continued beyond the session. They reported that: *Mam always comes out so relaxed – a new person after your treatment...she always looks forward to these relaxing sessions* (R6F) and *when you touched my partner, it made her feel that she wanted to come back to the hospice* (R29F).

Additionally, carers recognised that they were also being 'drawn into the treatments' and the treatment had a 'bystander effect', as described in Chapter 10. This may be due to the neurological responses that take place in the brain, which result in feelings of empathy (see Chapter 4).

One carer said that he *...wanted to be the patient* (R2M) and a second said that *We felt so relaxed just listening to your voice at the bedside* (R35F). A third carer was so impressed that she said *...that was amazing to watch... I would like some of that* (R13F).

Some carers will openly ask if the therapist will 'show them how to do it'. They feel that being able to contribute something to the wellbeing of their loved one would help them to cope, either at home or when a therapist isn't available in the hospital/hospice. After watching a loved one receive a HEARTS treatment, one female carer explained, *...I could cope a lot better at home, if there was something I could do* (R17F), and a second carer asked *...can you show me how to do that? You make Mum so calm; I want to do the same* (R19F).

Sometimes a carer can be reluctant to offer HEARTS for the patient. S/he may feel so stressed that to add one more activity to an existing long list of commitments would not be in his/her best interests. Additionally, there may be 'past history' in the relationship that makes HEARTS difficult to give, and in some situations, difficult to receive. However, as Case study 11.1 demonstrates, not all carers will want to participate in delivering HEARTS – and it is important that as therapists we remain non-judgemental about the carer's decision.

Case study 11.1. Restoring touch in relationships

Pauline had advanced cancer and was anxious to resume some intimacy with her partner, Jim, who was concerned about causing her harm due to extensive bone metastases and Pauline's rapid weight loss. The therapist was asked to 'go and see the couple' and to show them some of 'that gentle therapy you have been doing'. On entry to the room, it was clear that Pauline was seriously ill; she was very pale, and spoke very quietly to the therapist. The therapist explained HEARTS to Pauline and gained consent to demonstrate some of the HEARTS components. She explained the basics of HEARTS to Jim, and encouraged him to join in with the process. Jim did so, although very reluctantly. The therapist closed the session with some disappointment, although she noticed that a little colour had come back into Pauline's face. She reported back to the nurses, feeling quite despondent that she had not been able to do more. However, on the way back to the office, she went through the cafe area, to find Pauline and Jim sitting at a table drinking tea. Pauline said, 'I feel so much better. Thank you so much.' Jim expressed his thanks too, but the therapist later discovered that Pauline received complementary therapies to help address her need for touch until she died a few weeks later.

As the therapist had no prior relationship with the couple or knowledge of the case history apart from physical symptoms, she did not feel it was within her role to start inquiring as to why Jim did not want to be involved in the HEARTS Process. It may have been that he did not feel confident, he may have felt that he could disappoint his wife by not giving her what she really wanted, or he may have been uncomfortable with the approach. The therapist felt that she was right not to cross the boundary, and that she had done the best she could in the circumstances.

OPTIONS FOR LEARNING

There are three options of using HEARTS with carers. One is to encourage carers to receive a 'treat' for themselves, which can be given at the bedside if required. A second option is that where a carer feels motivated to give HEARTS to a loved one, the carer can be assisted in learning some of the basics of HEARTS. This is particularly useful as therapists cannot always be where they are needed, and it is helpful for carers to feel they have something that they can contribute. As one carer said to the therapist, ...*I could do that when you are not here* (R33F). The third option involves the patient in 'giving back' to the carer. Where a patient is cognitively and physically able, s/he may want to offer HEARTS to the carer as an expression of affection, gratitude, respect or simply something that they can share together. Sometimes patients may feel that therapies, or something that is potentially pleasant and enjoyable, are being given in a one-way direction, towards themselves; they may feel that their loved ones are 'missing out'. This reciprocal activity can restore touch where it has broken down. One carer said that ...*I really enjoyed the opportunity of being close to my husband in this way* (R10F) and a patient said ...*I enjoyed receiving HEARTS from my partner* (R10F). Additionally, in cases where touch had broken down between partners, practising HEARTS helped to restore the relationship, resulting in two marriages!

HELPING A CARER TO LEARN HEARTS

One of the really useful characteristics of HEARTS is that it is easy to learn, and most carers like to learn the strokedown, therapeutic holding and possibly some gentle palming. As more than one person can easily work with a patient at the same time, the Hands-on work lends itself to being 'copied', so the carer(s) can mirror the movements the therapist is demonstrating.

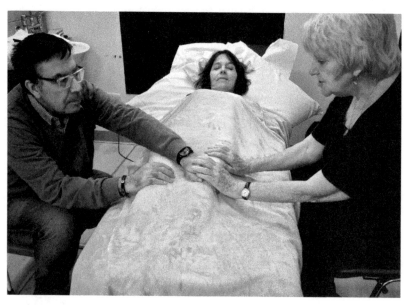

Figure 11.1. One of the best ways of teaching carers is for both therapist and carer to work with the patient at the same time

It is helpful to explain to the patient what will be happening during the 'training session' and for short periods of time the therapist will probably be more involved with the carer. Letting the patient know the process avoids him/her thinking that the carer and therapist are having their own conversation and ignoring the patient, who is a really important part of the process. It is always useful to ask for feedback from the patient, and this is a good way of involving him/her in the process.

The following case study demonstrates how learning HEARTS occurred through the carer working alongside the therapist.

Case study 11.2. Using HEARTS at home

Kathy was caring for her father Kevin at home. There was a strong bond between father and daughter, although Kathy was finding the caring role quite difficult as she also had her own family to care for. She had watched the nurse therapist carry out a HEARTS treatment for Kevin, and noticed how much more settled and relaxed he was after only a few minutes. The nurse therapist, Miriam, asked Kathy if she would like to learn some of the strokes so Kathy could use the approach when she was on her own. Kathy agreed, and Miriam suggested that Kathy could mirror what she was doing. Kathy was a little apprehensive at first, with questions such as: Was the pressure right? Was it too fast or too slow? How long should she do the towel stroking for? Could any other family members join in? Learning HEARTS was a meaningful turning point in Kevin's care as Kathy felt that she had a resource that she could use to help her father in a variety of situations.

An advantage of a carer learning HEARTS is that it takes the therapeutic approach outside the clinical setting and can form the basis of self-help. It is easy to see the carer as a person who is in the role of looking after a seriously ill partner, family member or friend. However, in the context of learning some aspects of the HEARTS approach that they particularly like, another side of their persona comes into play – that of the adult learner.

CHARACTERISTICS OF ADULT LEARNERS

When transferring a role from therapist to teacher, it may be helpful to have some awareness of the way adults learn. Remember that adult carers will:

- Want to learn something that is feasible and that they can use immediately.

- Have considerable life experience that forms a foundation for new material.

- Appreciate that the therapist is sharing their skills with them and will want to be involved.

- Have other commitments in their lives apart from the time s/he spends with the therapist.

- Expect their perceptions and experience to be respected.

- Appreciate constructive feedback.

- Want the efforts they make to be valued – by both the patient and the therapist.

(Daines, Daines and Graham 2002)

Additionally, adults will have preferred styles of learning. Kolb (1984) devised the original Learning Styles Inventory that was later adapted by Honey and Mumford (1992). In this model, four styles of learning were identified: activist, reflector, theorist and pragmatist. More details about the characteristics of each learning style are given below:

- Activists want to get on with the task. There is an urgency to learn as much as they can, and they will embrace HEARTS enthusiastically. They may need to slow down and reflect on how they are working with HEARTS; this is where feedback from the patient is helpful. Activists will enjoy working alongside a therapist and they will learn least from watching a demonstration from the bedside.

- Reflectors are likely to ask questions and to think about HEARTS before jumping in to learn new skills. They can get into detail and may start thinking of different ways of delivering HEARTS before they have learned the strokedown, for example. They like to hear about research and the experiences of others carers (if possible) and also the experiences of the patient. They will be more cautious than the activists, and may like to take time to think about how and when they want to learn – so a separate appointment may need to be made.

- Theorists like structured ways of working and may find the intuitive side of HEARTS something of a challenge. They like lectures (which are unlikely to happen in the context in which we work) and demonstrations. For these learners, the treatment that the therapist has offered to the patient may be sufficient to serve as a demonstration. Theorists will like notes that include some theoretical information. They may initially be guarded about learning something new, although they may be highly motivated to do so.

- Pragmatists like to set clear goals and need to be able to recognise a practical application (this is easy to do in the context of carer/patient care). They will be concerned with detail and dislike the theoretical aspects of a situation… but they do like a 'right answer'. They prefer a structured style of teaching and will be dissatisfied with unstructured activities where there is no clear purpose.

While HEARTS is easy to learn, no oil is applied, the patient is covered, and the touch is light and gentle, the rhythm being of importance, one problem that carers may encounter at home is to identify the best place to carry out a HEARTS treatment. Depending on the wellness of the patient, it may be easier to offer HEARTS with the patient seated in a chair or supported by pillows leaning against a table. The patient can still be covered with a favourite blanket, or the texture of a dressing gown may suffice. Another place for HEARTS at home is as part of personal care, to be carried out after washing or bathing, or when helping someone to rest.

RECOMMENDATIONS

- It is possible for more than one family member to work with a patient at a time, which could facilitate the involvement of other family members at the same time (see Chapter 6).

- Encourage a carer to have a treatment at the bedside. The patient may also benefit from watching, just as the carers benefit from watching the patient receive a treatment (see Chapter 12).

- Providing that the patient is able, encourage them to recall some of the aspects of HEARTS that they like for self-soothing.

- Do encourage carers or a family member to learn HEARTS, but remember that learning one more thing might be just too much for an individual.

- Don't be surprised if carers have a different learning style from yourself.

- It is helpful to have some background notes readily available.

- If you have already attended the two-day HEARTS therapists course, joining the HEARTS teachers' course may be something you would like to consider in the future.

SUMMARY

This chapter has reviewed the current training available for learning the practice of HEARTS and recommendations have been made for future development. The challenges that face carers have been discussed, together with carers' motivations to learn HEARTS for use when a therapist isn't available. Learning styles have been described, together with some consideration of the characteristics of adult learners. The principles discussed have been illustrated through case histories and recommendations have been suggested.

Chapter 12

THE THERAPISTS' PERSPECTIVES: RESULTS OF THE HEARTS PILOT SURVEY

INTRODUCTION

Since the early part of the 21st century, many research studies have been conducted to explore and examine the value and effectiveness, or otherwise, of complementary therapies. As HEARTS is a recent, innovative therapeutic approach, incorporating a variety of practices and principles, there are challenges in gathering evaluative data, as well as information about its integration within clinical practice. Published chapters, with illustrative case histories, have been described and explored within three complementary therapy textbooks: Carter and Mackereth (2017), Cawthorn and Mackereth (2010) and Mackereth and Carter (2006). A review of a palliative care complementary therapy service from 2012–14 reported on HEARTS sessions (*n*=114) with positive feedback, including 'loved it' and 'soothing, calming and relaxing' (Mackereth *et al.* 2016).

Since the inception of HEARTS, numerous case studies have been sent to the authors from both the one-day and two-day courses. The authors have provided informal mentoring and feedback about the reported practice, with carefully and sensitively anonymised case studies shared at training events, conference presentations and more recently, through publications. The case histories and practice of the therapies have been mainly positive and demonstrated good practice in working with vulnerable patients. The more challenging accounts often related to confidence issues and practical barriers in complex areas of practice, such as explaining the intervention to medical staff or offering HEARTS to patients with critical illness or where the patient's capacity to consent was difficult to ascertain.

In 2017, a questionnaire was drafted, with the assistance of a PhD-prepared researcher, which was piloted with eight experienced therapists attending a HEARTS teacher training course. As a result, minor adjustments were made to the final questionnaire based on the responses and feedback about the ease of completion. Both an electronic version and hard copies were distributed to individuals who had completed a HEARTS two-day course from a secure database. These contacts had expressed an interest in being kept informed of new courses and developments in HEARTS. A copy of the questionnaire and the letter sent to the therapists has been included in the Appendix of this book. A total of 38 past students voluntarily completed questionnaires, and these were returned within six months of distribution. However, due to likely changes in personal email addresses and changes of circumstances, it is not possible to confidently state the percentage response.

This chapter discusses the results of the questionnaire and explores some of the issues and reported experiences of the respondents (*n*=38) practising HEARTS in clinical, supportive and palliative care settings. Some questions allowed for a respondent (R) to give an additional comment; these are italicised and coded with a respondent number and stated gender, for example, R2M (male) or R3F (female). The analysis of the response includes reporting via tables of responses to given descriptors and thematic clustering of respondents' volunteered comments.

Questions 1 and 2. Demographic characteristics

From the questionnaire results, 36 females and 2 males practised HEARTS. Eighty-two per cent of the respondents were aged 51 (*n*=31) and over, with equal numbers in the 51–60 age range and the over-60s. Sixteen per cent (*n*=6) were aged between 41 and 50. Only one of the therapists (3%) was aged between 21 and 30, and none of the therapists was aged under 21.

Questions 3 and 4. Respondents' professional background prior to HEARTS training

In terms of professional training, 68 per cent (*n*=26) identified themselves as being complementary therapists and 29 per cent (*n*=11) reported that they were both healthcare professionals and complementary therapists. Only one respondent (3%) was a nurse who had not undertaken formal training in a complementary therapy. Of the 38 respondents, 20 (53%) had completed aromatherapy training and 20 (53%) had completed massage training. There may be some overlap with these two complementary therapies depending on the training establishment attended. Sometimes massage is included in the full aromatherapy course; in other situations, the student has to complete a separate massage qualification as a prerequisite to attending an aromatherapy course. Marginally, reflexology was the most common qualification; 22 (58%) of the group were reflexologists and 8 (21%) were Reiki practitioners. It needs to be acknowledged that some respondents had completed training in more than one therapy. Other modalities listed, but not necessarily practised, in a clinical setting were identified as relaxation, hypnotherapy, acupuncture, craniosacral therapy and Emmett (a muscle release therapy). Additionally, two therapists reported practising the 'M' technique, a modified form of massage therapy (Buckle 2003).

Question 5. Therapists' descriptors for HEARTS

Therapists were asked to choose three words from a list of 12 descriptors that they felt best described the HEARTS Process (see the Appendix). All 38 respondents answered this question; however, two respondents ringed only two of the words (see Table 12.1).

Table 12.1. Descriptors of HEARTS

	No of descriptors = 12	N=112 words, 98% response	Respondents, N=38
1	Compassionate	21 (19%)	55%
2	Calming	19 (17%)	50%
3	Soothing	13 (12%)	34%
4	Simplicity	13 (12%)	34%
5	'In the moment'	13 (12%)	34%
6	Peaceful	9 (8%)	24%
7	Effective	9 (8%)	24%
8	Powerful	8 (7%)	21%
9	Unconditional	4 (4%)	11%

cont.

10	Emotional	3 (3%)	8%
11	A 'reverie'	No response	0
12	Kind	No response	0

In addition to the prepared list, derived in part to responses to the pilot questionnaire, respondents were also asked to add their own perspective. Aside from the value to patients typified by the comment ...*relaxing and comforting – I hear this a lot in patient feedback* (R2M), the therapists valued the adaptability and the empathic nature of HEARTS, with statements such as:

Client-centred caring (R1F)

Adaptable to meet client's needs (R14F)

...individualised, meeting the...needs of the patient (R16F)

Empathic treatment (R12F)

One respondent added that HEARTS could be included within their existing therapy, being ...*encompassing of different therapies* (R5F). HEARTS was also judged to be:

...non-threatening, any time, any place, anywhere, always available (R18F)

...very unintrusive and can be done anywhere (R33F)

A number of respondents reported the intervention as a means of connecting. For example, one respondent stated, *I am here for you... now* (R19F), while others talked about the type of connection:

Empowering...there is an emotional connection (R10M)

A powerful connection with the client (R24F)

...the intimate power and effect of human touch (R29F)

HEARTS provides a means to connect with another person and hold them in a safe place (R34F)

Finally, one respondent acknowledged all of the descriptors listed and added, ...*it is all of the above and it works* (R15F).

Question 6. Views on benefits for patients

Table 12.2 lists the respondents' assessments of benefit to patients, utilising the given descriptors. Additional comments highlighted that many of the descriptors were relevant to their experience, typified by the statements: ...*really, all of the above* (R17F) and ...*I could have circled all of these words* (R33F).

Respondents added their own perspectives of the benefits of HEARTS as ...*empowering to patient – an oasis of calm in chaos* (R1F) and providing *feelings of peace and tranquillity* (R16F). One respondent implied that HEARTS could possibly assist with resilience by suggesting the intervention ...*allows a person to regain balance and store* (R34F). Another respondent stated, ...*also, promotes a bond between therapist and client which enhances the initial treatment* (R25F).

Finally, one respondent widened the view of benefits to patients by including carers, recommending, *Simple tips may be taught to carers for home use and is then beneficial to the giver and receiver* (R14F).

Table 12.2. Descriptors of benefits for patients

	No of descriptors = 12	N=114 words, 100% response	Respondents, N=38
1	Calms	25 (22%)	66%
2	Reduces anxiety	24 (21%)	63%
3	Relaxes	19 (17%)	50%
4	Enhances wellbeing	12 (11%)	32%
5	Soothes	8 (7%)	21%
6	Promotes trust	6 (5%)	16%
7	Feels comforted	6 (5%)	16%
8	Reduces tension	4 (4%)	11%
9	Eases pain	4 (4%)	11%
10	Feels valued	2 (2%)	5%
11	Promotes sleep	2 (2%)	5%
12	Provides enjoyment	2 (2%)	5%

Question 7. Therapists' reported gains from HEARTS

Therapists were asked to select three words from a list of ten that best described how a therapist gains from working with HEARTS, and these choices are listed in Table 12.3. Safety and simplicity merits were acknowledged in the following:

To witness the merits of 'less is more' (R3F)

...being able to offer a therapy in spite of any patient problems (R18F)

...being able to provide an effective therapy when other therapies may not be appropriate (R20F)

...the bond between therapist and patient is enhanced, which I feel is also described by tuning in to the patient (R25F)

Additionally, the theme of connection was raised again in responses to this question:

Allows me to reach out to a person and help them to feel loved (R34F)

A connection with your patient (R16F)

Table 12.3. Therapists' advantages of using HEARTS

	No of descriptors = 10	N=112 words, 98% response	Respondents, N=38
1	Able to tune into the patient	36 (32%)	95%
2	Able to offer a skilled intervention	22 (20%)	58%
3	Calming	15 (13%)	39%
4	Being in the moment	14 (13%)	37%
5	Relaxing to do	10 (9%)	26%
6	Being a resource	8 (7%)	21%
7	Feels grounded	6 (5%)	16%
8	Enjoyment	2 (2%)	5%
9	Develops confidence	1 (0.9%)	3%
10	Feels refreshed	1 (0.9%)	3%

Question 8. Rationale for not providing or offering HEARTS

Given the claimed safety and adaptability of HEARTS for a range of healthcare settings, therapists were asked to identify and report three situations when they decided not to offer HEARTS. Thirteen therapists did not give a response to this question, either leaving the space blank, or writing 'not appropriate' or 'not relevant' or 'nothing yet'. In total, there were 32 responses. One therapist wrote that she could not think of any situation as: *You can always use some aspect of HEARTS no matter what the situation or place* (R8F).

Consent concerns

For 25 respondents, consent was cited as the major issue blocking an offer to provide HEARTS. Eleven respondents made statements related to consent, and these included patients who refused HEARTS or who appeared not to want the offered intervention:

> *Patient not open to any form of complementary therapy* (R9F)

> *The patient not liking or wanting touch (R26F)*

> *Patient reluctant to try HEARTS* (R26F)

Respondents did give more, somewhat distressing, detail related to this decision:

> *The patient was in extreme pain and did not want any intervention (R23F)*

and

> *...a young man had a fear of dying in the treatment* (R6F)

The following are statements that relate to possible cognitive impairment, including:

> *Dementia, the patient did not understand and a second patient was very confused about his/her surroundings* (R12F)

> *and the...patient was drifting in and out of consciousness* (R1F)

One respondent reported that one patient was ...*unable* to fully consent (R23F) but did not give a reason, with another stating that ...*a mental health condition* (R17F) prevented assurance of consent.

Two therapists said that although a patient may refuse initially, they would keep in contact and seek to earn the patient's trust.

Challenging and blocking situations

Respondents made statements about challenging situations that had blocked them from offering HEARTS, and these included ...*working in a noisy busy ward or bay* (R5F) and when there were ...*many people in the home – both family and healthcare professionals at the same time* (R16F).

Two respondents mentioned not having sufficient time – first, to offer it in the first place: [I was] *in a rush* (10R) and second, to always give it ...*in conjunction with reflexology* (R25F).

Five respondents felt that there could be a lack *of understanding* on the part of patients of what was being offered. One respondent reported that ...*one patient had fixed ideas of what therapists do* (R17F).

For some therapists, HEARTS was either no longer offered or stopped when a patient became *restless* (R27F). Additionally, therapists did not raise HEARTS as an option with a patient who had ...*cognitive impairment* (no detail given) (R7F) and with another patient with ...*severe depression* (R10F). One respondent stated the ...*patient's personal reasons* (not disclosed) as a concern that was blocking an offer of HEARTS (R18F). Another respondent stated a patient was *deaf* and did not appear to be ...*wanting touch* (R36F).

Two respondents mentioned patient preference for ...*massage* due to ...*cultural difference* (R36F), with *language difficulties* raised by another as a concern blocking an offer of HEARTS (R36F).

Finally, two respondents mentioned *confidence*. First, one therapist did not *feel confident* in her skills (R2F), while a second therapist stated that the patient ...*didn't have enough confidence in her* (R17).

Question 9. Suggested 'appropriate' uses for HEARTS

Therapists were asked to report up to three situations where they thought HEARTS was the most appropriate treatment at the time. Table 12.4 summarises data from the responses and also gives details about observed responses. There was concern about 'traditional' complementary therapies, which included massage, aromatherapy and reflexology being perhaps too invasive, with HEARTS being of particular value with patients who were anxious, agitated and at end of life.

Table 12.4. Appropriate use of HEARTS

Situations	N=51*	Examples of therapists' comments
To help alleviate anxiety/panic/agitation	16 (31%)	*Patient awaiting results of scans* (R8F) *Female patient having panic attack* (R13F) *Very anxious and upset patient... and anxious carer* (R14F) *Patient unable to focus on anything but prognosis – much calmer after treatment* (R17F)
Traditional complementary therapies (CTs) were not appropriate	11 (22%)	*Not appropriate [when] patients not open to CTs [so] have used HEARTS when I can't use other CTs* (R9F) *A way of opening interest in caring touch* (R10F) *Concerned about massage as patient was easily bruised* (R12F) *Well-intentioned touch and holding useful in the first instance* (R25F) Where *something really simple was required* (R27F) *Patient had a deep vein thrombosis and would not agree to reflexology* (R20F) *Reflexology not wanted* (R25F) *Skin too tender to use oil* (R17F) *When light touch was indicated* (R35F) *Patient was very weary with low energy* (R38F)
End of life/fear of dying/dying phase	8 (16%)	*Very gentle and effective therapy at this stage (R21)* *Patient very fragile, limited amount of time – patient found it very beneficial* (R28F)

cont.

Situations	N=51*	Examples of therapists' comments
Emotional upset	4 (8%)	*Patient soothed by being wrapped in a blanket* (R4F) *Cognitive impairment had left the patient angry and frustrated* (R7F) *Patient exhausted and needed to sleep* (R26F) *Patient had been given bad news* (R13F)
Extreme pain	3 (6%)	*Below knee amputation with phantom limb pain – pain-free after HEARTS* (R17F) *Patient in pain and needed some space in which to relax* (R32F)
Extra cover needed	3 (6%)	*Patient in a cold area* (R2F) *Elderly palliative care patient did not want to be uncovered* (R23F) *Patient very cold and treatment given through two duvets – did not want hands/feet exposed* (R14F)
Body image	2 (4%)	No additional comment (R4F)
Infection	1 (2%)	No additional comment (R3F)
Cachexia	1 (2%)	No additional comment (R3F)
Breathlessness	1 (2%)	*Embarrassment* (R4F)
Tension	1 (2%)	*Patient didn't think it would help but relaxed and slept* (R38F)

* More than one situation was reported by respondents.

Question 10. Reported 'bystander effects' and patient responses to HEARTS

Therapists were asked to report up to three examples of unsolicited feedback from a family member/carer present during HEARTS treatment. Sometimes the carer reportedly benefited directly from watching the treatment taking place. Just as the 'bystanders' were entranced by watching the treatments at a complementary therapy exhibition, described earlier in Chapter 1, so carers/family members watching a patient receiving a HEARTS treatment can be drawn into the process. Before discussing the data, I would like to comment that the act of reading and collating the data triggered a 'feel good' response. Perhaps these accounts created imagined scenarios for the reader, an example of a 'secondary bystander effect'. It is important to acknowledge that watching someone receiving other forms of complementary therapy treatments may also trigger a relaxation response in bystanders, and a desire to receive the treatment themselves.

Observations of patients' responses to HEARTS

In total, there were 23 comments reporting observer feedback; importantly, these are recalled rather than verbatim comments. The observers were largely family members visiting the patient, although there were comments attributed to staff members.

Relaxation was a common observer comment: ...*he has calmed down* (R27F) and ...*she looks so relaxed* (R38F). Some carers went beyond this with comments suggesting effects on wellbeing, such as:

I've never seen her so relaxed...it really calms her...you take such good care of her (R1F)

Your touch made her feel safe (R34F)

He looks so relaxed...that looks so comforting (R3F)

It's like stroking a fretful child – calms them down (R23F)

He has fallen asleep – I have never seen him so relaxed since his diagnosis (R4F)

Two respondents reported carers' comments that implied effects beyond one session:

Mam comes out so relaxed – a new person after your treatment (R6F)

[She] always looks forward to these relaxing session...when you touched my partner it made her feel that she wanted to come back to the hospice (R29F)

'Bystander effects' from observing HEARTS

The respondents reported comments made by observers that were linked to the observers' emotional and physical responses to watching a HEARTS treatment; they suggest a change of state for the carer. One therapist said that the carer ...*wanted to be the patient* (R2M).

Three responses referred directly to the *relaxing* effects on the observers. First, one visitor said, *I can't believe how deeply relaxed I feel too* (R5F); second, another relative said, *...watching makes me relaxed as well* (R18F); and third, one respondent observed, *...it was relaxing [for him/her] just to watch...the relative looked calmer and less anxious* (R21F). HEARTS includes the therapeutic use of the voice; this had also impacted on the patient's visitors, with one reportedly saying, *...we felt relaxed just listening to your voice at the bedside* (R35F).

Two respondents made links with effects on the carer from observing the treatment; first, one carer said, *It's so comforting to see my partner so relaxed... It looks very peaceful* (R30F). Another carer recognised an effect on her own wellbeing linked to watching HEARTS: *...I feel so much better having seen mum calmed down after your treatment* (R19F) and a staff member said *I nearly fell asleep... That was amazing* (R6F).

Two observers at the bedside were reported to have said how ... *surprised* (R26F) they were that something *...so simple could have such an effect* (R38F). One carer, hinting perhaps that she wished to learn the technique, was reported to have said *...it appears easy to do* (R33F). Finally, one carer was reportedly so impressed that she said, *That was amazing to watch...I would like some of that* (R13F).

Therapists' stories

The following accounts of outcomes from the carer's perspective were reported:

A family member was *tearful and grateful* for the peace that had been given to her husband (R8F)

The carer of a young man was tearful at the end of the treatment as she was *overwhelmed* by the peace that HEARTS had brought to her son (R8F)

A family member joined in by listening and said she felt *very soothed* and more relaxed than ever (R17F)

One man saw his wife receive HEARTS and described it as one of the most *beautiful things* he had seen (R28F)

I carried out a treatment on a very agitated woman. At the end of the treatment the patient, carer and son were all asleep (R34F)

Relatives told me that just watching calmed them down and reduced their anxiety (R35F)

The carer was touched by love and kindness shown to their loved one (R28)

Staff look forward to my presence – individuals were calmer, more reasonable and looked forward to the treatment (R11F)

Carers learning to do HEARTS

Words from carers:

Thank you, I feel I can do something to help my partner (R4F)

That is so simple and easy to do for each other (R4F)

I really appreciated the opportunity of being close to my husband in this way (R10F)

I enjoyed receiving HEARTS from my partner (R10F)

Show me how so we can do it for each other (R13F)

It looks simple enough that I could do it (R18F)

Can you show me how to do that? You make Mum so calm – I want to do the same (R19F)

Can I do that? (R27F)

I could do that when you are not here (R33)

A partner asked to learn HEARTS and said she could cope at home if she could help in this way (R17F)

HEARTS empowered a carer in a situation where she felt helpless before (R16F)

Therapists' stories of learning:

A carer said it was easy to learn and she wanted to do it at home for her partner (R26F)

A carer was happy to learn HEARTS and to be able to help her partner (R26F)

Learning HEARTS was beneficial to the patient and was also calming and therapeutic for the carer (R35F)

The patient's wife was keen to learn all aspects of HEARTS as she could see the calming effects. She was caring 24 hours a day and felt it would be useful (R8F)

I have shown family members how to use the 'strokedown' – others are just too stressed (R9F)

All the carers I have worked with have been very enthusiastic to try any measures which will calm and soothe the people for whom they are caring (R11F)

Teaching a partner how to do HEARTS led to a resumption of a much more intimate relationship and resulted in a wedding! (R35F)

Question 11. Unexpected patients' responses to HEARTS

Following accounts of unexpected responses to HEARTS from the pilot questionnaire ($n=8$), therapists, in the final version of the questionnaire, were asked to describe any unexpected reactions to receiving a HEARTS treatment. Of these respondents ($n=29$), 20 made comments about unexpected reactions.

Eight therapists identified an unexpected emotional reaction, such as crying or laughing. Of these eight respondents, four acknowledged that patients may experience much pleasure, but can become very emotional. One of these therapists reported that a patient had cried, but had felt better for the release of tension. One said that a patient had remained agitated and another had become restless. A third therapist reported a case of using imagery that was chosen by the patient which evoked painful memories (see Chapter 7).

One therapist reported bodily noises emitting from the patients, including passing flatus, snorting and snoring, all of which may have caused the individual embarrassment.

Two therapists reported that they had not observed any adverse reactions – just 'calm, peace and pleasure'. A further two therapists perceived that by 'an unexpected reaction', the question implied crying, which is not necessarily a 'bad' reaction.

Of the remainder, two therapists reported patients' spontaneous experiences of visual imagery concerned with colours that were not reportedly initiated by the therapist. Both experiences were enjoyed and calmed patients; one of the patients found the experience very *uplifting*. This is not an infrequent experience when patients become deeply relaxed.

One patient enjoyed HEARTS so much that she wanted it outside the hospice and would not accept any other therapeutic approach.

Patients who had received several kinds of massage return to HEARTS over and over again.

One report was of pain relief for a young man with extreme abdominal tension. Gentle holding enabled tension release that had a profound and beneficial effect on his pain. Patients are surprised by how something as simple as towel stroking can create such profound calm and peace.

A female patient had been refused massage at one support centre; her medical practitioner did not recommend massage treatment. HEARTS was used with profound effects for both the patient and the therapist.

Question 12. Environmental constraints in the workplace

Constraints were varied and are discussed below. It was encouraging that 11 of the respondents did not raise concerns about environmental and other restrictions, with a further two respondents leaving the question unanswered. Noise was the main constraint reported. It was reported by nine respondents, who were mainly working on hospital wards. These respondents associated the noise as coming from everyday ward activities. One therapist reported that there was a toilet across the hallway from the treatment area, and it is likely that there were frequent sounds linked to interruptions of people using the facilities, such as doors closing and the toilet being flushed.

As therapists, it is important to distance ourselves from environmental distractions (except for emergencies such as fire alarms!). Often we can become determined to create a 'therapeutic space' for patients, and in this pursuit, we inevitably become frustrated by environmental and noise pollution in the real world of clinical care. Therapists who have worked in hospitals, hospices and even in a patient's home come to accept that we cannot exert the same controls as we would in a private therapy space or spa. Interruptions such as telephones ringing, staff communicating, patients having bedside treatments and tea trolleys are all part of working in clinical spaces. Importantly, patients may not feel able or comfortable about complaining about the intrusive sounds of healthcare business. Certainly, staff are likely to develop a greater tolerance, given that these environments are their workplaces, and they are likely to be absorbed in care delivery with noise becoming normalised over time. All of us can seek to reduce unnecessary noise and interruptions, but a realistic response to inevitable noise and interruptions is to say to the patient, 'You may be aware of background sounds and interruptions, but while I am providing HEARTS, you may or may not notice these sounds. It is just the ward staff going about the place, doing their job, or visitors may be talking to their loved ones...bring your awareness back to listening to my voice, my hands, the soft comfort of the blanket on your legs, your body and your arms...' (see Chapter 5 for further suggestions for managing interruptions and noise).

Eight respondents questioned the suitability of the treatment space and the need to negotiate around pieces of clinical equipment as a concern and a constraint. One therapist identified the proximity of other patients as being potentially intrusive; three commented about working in a chemotherapy suite and the infusion devices/ delivery systems attached to patients. Two respondents discussed working in a patient's home, with the ability to deliver treatment hampered by furniture and with the patient being seated on a chair. One respondent identified difficulty in treating a patient who was positioned in the middle of double bed; in this position the patient was difficult to reach comfortably. Therapists need to be comfortable while delivering the treatment; when possible, a patient may be required to change his/her position or to be moved in reach of the therapist. The latter requires moving and handling training and additional equipment and staff resources. The other option is for the therapist to modify the treatment to accommodate the limitations of the situation. It is important to acknowledge, given the feedback from patients in this study and elsewhere (Mackereth *et al.* 2016), that HEARTS can have profound effects even when it may seem to the therapist that it was not 'good enough'. Partly, this may be a desire to make the session perfect and also possibly an under-estimation of how welcome and valued the session was to the patient.

Five therapists reported that there were variations in the ex-pectations of clinical staff and patients, with typical comments indicating an expectation of an oiled massage or a more traditional complementary therapy, such as reflexology. Two of these respondents said that sometimes the voiced expectations of staff influenced their motivation to offer HEARTS. Additionally, they suggested that there was a need for some education of clinical staff, which would help to increase awareness of the potential benefits of HEARTS to patients.

Five reported time constraints, one therapist saying she was required to see a minimum of five patients in her working day (hours were not specified) for existing therapies. This would suggest that HEARTS was an 'add-on' or in addition to scheduled referrals. Another comment was that one nurse found it difficult to fit HEARTS sessions within her nursing duties, and added that she would like to see a complementary therapist employed full time.

Two respondents said that staff interruptions and comments on the treatments from other healthcare professionals observing in the locality was distracting. Typically comments included, 'That looks good' or 'We could all do with some of that.' On face value, one could view these comments as intrusive, but they may also be perceived as encouraging as they appear to draw positive attention to the treatment. A talk on HEARTS to staff, to include a demonstration on one of the staff members, may be helpful. Readers will probably agree that receiving a therapy is often the best way to understand and evaluate it. As mentioned earlier, patients receiving HEARTS may be oblivious to other people's comments – it is perhaps advisable to simply acknowledge the staff's comments non-verbally, with a nod and a smile, and continue to pay attention to the patient and the delivery of the treatment. One respondent commented that every staff member appeared to be both supportive and encouraging about the use of HEARTS with patients. Perhaps this suggests how visually powerful HEARTS is to observe, and how this might help to promote the intervention.

LIMITATIONS

Accessing respondents was challenging given that participants may have worked temporarily or part time, either as paid staff or as volunteers in healthcare settings. An institutional ethical review of any study and access approval from managers of complementary therapy services to distribute questionnaires would be required to complete a formal larger-scale survey. Another option considered for data collection was telephone or face-to-face interviews, but this was discounted as the project did not have the funds or other resources to conduct these activities. It is important to state that the sample was self-selecting and cannot be generalised to the wider population of HEARTS practitioners. Importantly, our respondents were therapists and/or health professionals, and we did not have direct feedback from patients and carers.

CONCLUSIONS

We recommend that future research work seeks to capture the experiences and responses of those who receive the therapy. Given that the largest area of clinical practice is with patients in supportive and palliative care, such projects are challenging but possible, particularly if outcome measures and data collection techniques are not complex or burdensome. Longer-term outcomes would require a study population that might be living with a chronic illness. Some of these diseases have periods of exacerbation or remission, for example multiple sclerosis; such variables would need to be considered in any study design. In supporting greater integration of HEARTS, evaluation data is necessary to provide information to those that fund services and costs associated with training of therapists and health professionals. It is important to acknowledge that HEARTS does not require special equipment, such as massage and essential oils, and can be done in clinical settings in a relatively short period of time. As the pool of therapists trained in HEARTS expands, it is likely that researchers in supportive and palliative care will become aware of its increasing usage. As part of informing health professionals, therapists and researchers, an important recommendation is for HEARTS practitioners to share their work through publishing case studies and sharing their experiences at conferences and workshops.

APPENDIX

LETTER CIRCULATED WITH
THE QUESTIONNAIRE
May 2017

Phone:
Email:

Dear HEARTS therapists

I am writing to ask for your help in finding out how the HEARTS Process is being used in practice. I am writing a book about HEARTS that will be published in 2018; its provisional title is *Touch and Relaxation Skills in Cancer Care: The HEARTS Process*, and it will be published by Singing Dragon. The results from the questionnaires will be used in the book, possibly in a discussion chapter about the potential for integrating HEARTS into supportive care in acute and hospice environments.

The questionnaire is only two sides and it doesn't take long to complete. If you would like to add anything in the way of comments or case histories on a separate sheet, the information would be most useful. Please don't include any personal details about patients, as this data must remain confidential.

There are two ways of returning the questionnaire to me – either you can post the completed questionnaire to my home address: _____
or you can email it to me at: _____
I appreciate it won't be anonymous if you email it to me, so I am printing out the questionnaires as soon as they arrive and putting them straight into a file. Once they are in the file, they will be anonymous as I will add the paper copies to the file as well.

Please could you send the questionnaire back to me by 1 September 2017.

Do get in touch with me if you have any queries at all. If you know anyone who is using HEARTS, please would you forward this front sheet and the questionnaire to them.

I look forward to hearing from you, and thank you very much for your help.

All good wishes

Ann Carter, Complementary Therapies in Cancer Care

QUESTIONNAIRE: THE HEARTS PROCESS

1. Are you male/female? Please tick the appropriate box

    ☐ Male
    ☐ Female

2. What is your age range? Please tick the appropriate box

    ☐ Under 20
    ☐ 21–30
    ☐ 31–40
    ☐ 41–50
    ☐ 51–60
    ☐ Over 60
    ☐ Other

3. Please tick your professional training(s)

    ☐ Healthcare professional
    ☐ Complementary therapist
    ☐ Something else

    If 'something else', please state what the training was (e.g. teaching, administration): _____

4. Which two complementary therapies do you normally practise?

    ☐ Aromatherapy
    ☐ Massage
    ☐ Reflexology
    ☐ Reiki
    ☐ Something else

    If 'something else', please state what the therapy(s) are: _____

    _____

5. Please circle up to three of the following words that best describe the HEARTS Process:

compassionate	calming	emotional
soothing	simplicity	effective
powerful	peaceful	a 'reverie'
'in the moment'	kind	unconditional

Your own word(s): _____

6. How do you think a patient benefits from receiving HEARTS? Please circle up to three of the following:

calms	relaxes	soothes
promotes sleep	provides enjoyment	enhances trust
eases pain	reduces anxiety	reduces tension
relieves discomfort	improves wellbeing	

Your own word(s): _____

7. What do you think a therapist gains from providing a HEARTS intervention? Please circle up to three of the following:

    feels grounded   relaxing to do   enjoyment

    calming   being a resource   develops
                                                 confidence

    able to offer a   feels refreshed   being 'in the
    skilled intervention   moment'

    able to 'tune in' to
    the patient

    Your own word(s): _____

8. Are there any situations where you decided not to offer HEARTS? Please give up to three examples:

    1. _____
    2. _____
    3. _____

9. Briefly describe up to three situations when you felt that offering HEARTS was the right choice to make:

    1. _____
    2. _____
    3. _____

10. If you have carried out any treatments for a patient where a family member/carer was present, please tell us up to three examples of any unsolicited feedback you may have received:

    1. _____
    2. _____
    3. _____

11. Have any of your patients experienced any unexpected reactions to HEARTS? If so, please tell what they were – up to three examples:

    1. _____
    2. _____
    3. _____

12. Are there any environmental or institutional constraints in your workplace, e.g. space, opinions of other staff, time allowed? Please state up to three constraints:

    1. _____
    2. _____
    3. _____

Thank you very much for your help.

If you would like to add anything on a separate sheet, your information would be very welcome.

REFERENCES

Argyle, M. (1975) *Bodily Communication*. New York: Routledge.

Arroyo-Anlló, E.M., Díaz, J.P. and Gil, R. (2013) 'Familiar music as an enhancer of self-consciousness in patients with Alzheimer's disease.' *BioMed Research International*. Available at www.hindawi.com/journals/bmri/2013/752965/

Autton, N. (1989) *Touch: An Exploration*. London: Darton, Longman & Todd.

Battino, R. (2000) *Guided Imagery and Other Approaches to Healing*. Bancyfelin: Crown House Publishing.

Bellis, M.A., Hughes, K., Leckenby, N., Perkins, C. and Lowey, H. (2014) 'National Household Survey of adverse childhood experiences and their relationship with resilience to health-harming behaviors in England.' *BMC Medicine 12*, 72, 1–10.

Bertolucci, L.F. (2011) 'Pandiculation: Nature's way of maintaining the functional integrity of the myofascial system.' *Journal of Bodywork and Movement 15*, 3, 268–280.

Betts, T. (1996) 'The fragrant breeze: The role of aromatherapy in treating epilepsy.' *Aromatherapy Quarterly 51*, 25–27.

Bloom, E. (2017) 'Prehabilitation: Evidence and Insight Review.' Available at www.macmillan.org.uk/_images/prehabilitation-evidence-and-insight-review_tcm9-335025.pdf

Booth, K., Maguire, P.M., Butterworth, T. and Hiller, V.F. (1996) 'Perceived professional support and the use of blocking behaviors by hospice nurses.' *Journal of Advanced Nursing 24*, 3, 522–527.

Bro, M.L., Jespersen, K.V., Hansen, B., Vuust, A., Abildgaard, N., Gram, J. and Johansen, C. (2017) 'Kind of blue: A systematic review and meta-analysis of music interventions in cancer treatment.' *Psychoncology 27*, 2, 386–400. Available at https://onlinelibrary.wiley.com/doi/full/10.1002/pon.4470

Buckle, J. (2003) *Clinical Aromatherapy: Essential Oils in Practice*. New York: Churchill Livingstone.

Burnham, M.M., Goodlin Jones, B., Gaylor, E.E. and Anders, T.F. (2002) 'Night time sleep-wake patterns and self-soothing from birth to one year of age: A longitudinal intervention study.' *Journal of Child Psychology and Psychiatry 43*, 6, 713–725.

Burton, N. (2015) 'Empathy vs sympathy.' *Psychology Today*, May 22. Available at www.psychologytoday.com/us/blog/hide-and-seek/201505/empathy-vs-sympathy

Bushdid, C., Magnasco, M.O., Vosshall, L.B. and Keller, A. (2014) 'Humans can discriminate more than 1 trillion olfactory stimuli.' *Science 343*, 618, 1379–1372.

Campbell, G. and Knowles, R. (2016) 'Caring for Carers.' In A. Carter and P.A. Mackereth (eds) *Aromatherapy, Massage and Relaxation in Cancer Care: An Integrative Resource for Practitioners (pp.196–209)*. London: Singing Dragon.

Canevelli, M., Valletta, M., Trebbastoni, A., Sarli, G., *et al.* (2016) 'Sundowning in dementia: Clinical relevance, pathophysiological determinants and therapeutic approaches.' *Frontiers in Medicine 3*, 73.

Carter, A. (2006) 'The HEARTS Process: Combining Therapeutic Approaches for Relaxation.' In P.A. Mackereth and A. Carter (eds) *Massage and Bodywork: Adapting Therapies for Cancer Care* (pp.123–136). London: Elsevier.

Carter, A. (2016) 'The HEARTS Process.' In A. Carter and P.A. Mackereth (eds) *Aromatherapy, Massage and Relaxation in Cancer Care: An Integrative Resource for Practitioners* (pp.167–180). London: Singing Dragon.

Carter, A. and Mackereth, P.A. (2006) *Massage and Bodywork: Adapting Therapies for Cancer Care*. London: Elsevier.

Carter, A. and Mackereth, P.A. (2010) 'Recognizing and Integrating "Hypnotic Trance" within "Touch Therapy" Work.' In A. Cawthorn and P.A. Mackereth (eds) *Integrative Hypnotherapy: Complementary Approaches in Clinical Care* (pp.115–128). London: Elsevier.

Carter, A. and Mackereth, P.A. (2017) 'The Resourceful Therapist.' In A. Carter and P.A. Mackereth (eds) *Aromatherapy, Massage and Relaxation in Cancer Care: An Integrative Resource for Practitioners* (pp.48–58). London: Singing Dragon.

Catani, M. (2017) 'A little man of some importance.' *Brain 140*, 11, 3055–3061.

Cawthorn, A. (2006) 'Working with the Denied Body.' In P.A. Mackereth and A. Carter (eds) *Massage and Bodywork: Adapting Therapies for Cancer Care* (pp.67–83). London: Elsevier.

Cawthorn, A. and Mackereth, P.A. (2010) *Integrated Hypnotherapy: Complementary Approaches in Clinical Care*. London: Elsevier.

Cawthorn, A. and Shepherd, B. (2010) 'Working with the Therapeutic Relationship.' In A. Cawthorn and P.A. Mackereth (eds) *Integrative Hypnotherapy: Complementary Approaches in Clinical Care* (pp.65–81). London: Elsevier.

Charalambous, A., Giannakopoulou, M., Bozas, E., Marcou, Y., Kitsios, P. and Paikousis, L. (2016) 'Guided imagery and progressive muscle relaxation as a cluster of symptoms management intervention in patients receiving chemotherapy: A randomized control trial.' *PLoS One 11*, 6. Available at www.ncbi.nlm.nih.gov/pubmed/27341675

Cheng, C.D., Volk, A.A. and Marini, Z.A. (2011) 'Supporting fathering through infant massage.' *Journal of Perinatal Education 20*, 4, 200–209.

Clark, A. (2010) 'Empathy and sympathy: Distinct directions in counseling.' *Journal of Mental Health Counseling 32*, 2, 95–101.

Cocksedge, S., George, B., Renwick, S. and Chew-Graham, C.A. (2013) 'Touch in primary care consultations: Qualitative investigations of doctors' and patients' perception.' *British Journal of General Practice 63*, 283–290.

Concise Oxford English Dictionary (2006) Oxford: Oxford University Press.

Cunico, L., Sartori, R., Marognoli, O. and Meneghini, A. (2012) 'Developing empathy in nursing students.' *Journal of Clinical Nursing 21*, 13–14, 2016–2025.

Daines, J.W., Daines, C. and Graham, B. (2002) *Adult Learning, Adult Teaching*. Cardiff: Welsh Academic Press.

Duhamel, G. (1919) *The Heart's Domain*. Brooks, NY: Eleanor Stimson Publishers.

Engel, B. (2008) 'What is compassion and how can it change my life?' *Psychology Today*, 29 April. Available at www.psychologytoday.com

Ferber, S.G., Feldman, R. and Makhoul, I.R. (2008) 'The development of maternal touch across the first year of life.' *Early Human Development 84*, 6, June, 363–370.

Field, T. (2014) *Touch* (2nd edn). Cambridge, MA: The MIT Press.

Field, T., Harding, J., Soliday, D.B. and Lasco, N. (1994) 'Touching in infant, toddler, and preschool nurseries.' *Early Child Development and Care 98*, 1, 113–120.

Forward, J.B., Greuter, N.E., Crisall, S.J. and Lester, H.F. (2015) 'Effect of structured touch and guided imagery for pain and anxiety in elective joint replacement patients: A randomized controlled trial.' *M-TIJRP: The Permanente Journal 19*, 4, 18–28.

Frank, D.A., Klass, P.E., Earls, F. and Eisenberg, L. (1996) 'Infants and young children in orphanages: One view from pediatrics and child psychiatry.' *Pediatrics 97*, 4, 569–578.

Gallese, V. (2003) 'The roots of empathy.' *Psychopathology 36*, 4, 171–180.

Gallese, V., Fadiga, L., Fogassi, L. and Rizzolatti, G. (1996) 'Action recognition in the premotor cortex.' *Brain 119*, 2, 593–609.

García, A.M., Ramón-Bou, N. and Porta, M. (2010) 'Isolated and joint effects of tobacco and alcohol consumption on risk of Alzheimer's disease.' *Journal of Alzheimer's Disease 20*, 2, 577–586.

Giacobbi, P.R., Stabler, M., Stewart, J., Jaeschke, A.M., Siebert, J.L. and Kelley, G.A. (2015) 'Guided imagery for arthritis and other rheumatic diseases: A systematic review of randomized controlled trials.' *Pain Management Nursing: Official Journal of the American Society of Pain Management Nurses 16*, 5, 792–803.

Gindrat, A.D., Chrytiris, M., Balerna, M., Rouiller, E. and Ghosh, A. (2015) 'Use-dependent cortical processing from fingertips in touchscreen phone users.' *Current Biology 25*, 1, 109–116.

Goldschmidt, B. and van Meines, N. (2012) *Comforting Touch in Dementia and End of Life Care*. Philadelphia, PA: Singing Dragon.

Guzzo, K.B. (2011) 'New fathers' experiences with their own fathers and attitudes towards fathering.' *Fathering 9*, 3, 268–290.

Hackman, E., Tomlinson, L., Mehrez, A. and Mackereth, P.A. (2013) 'Reducing patient distress: A CALM model for dementia care.' *British Journal of Nursing 222*, 4, S13-4, S16-8.

Handley, M., Bunn, F. and Goodman, C. (2017) 'Dementia-friendly interventions to improve the care of people living with dementia admitted to hospitals: A realist review.' *British Medical Journal Open 7*, 7.

Herz, R. (2009) 'Aroma facts and fictions: A scientific analysis of olfactory effects on mood, physiology and behaviour.' *International Journal of Neuroscience 119*, 2, 263–292.

Honey, P. and Mumford, A. (1992) *The Manual of Learning Styles.* Maidenhead: Peter Honey.

Jeffrey, D. (2016) 'Empathy, sympathy and compassion in health care: Is there a problem? Is there a difference? Does it matter?' *Journal of the Royal Society of Medicine 109*, 12, 446–452.

Jorgenson, J. (1996) 'The therapeutic use of companion animals in health care.' *Journal of Nursing Scholarship 29*, 3, 249–254.

King, K. (2010) 'A review of the effects of guided imagery on cancer patients with pain.' *Complementary Health Practice Review 15*, 2, 98–107.

Knight, S. (2002) *NLP at Work: The Difference that Makes a Difference in Business.* London: Nicholas Brealey Publishing. [First published 1995.]

Kolb, D.A. (1984) *Experiential Learning.* Upper Saddle River, NJ: Prentice Hall.

Leboyer, F. (1976) *Loving Hands: The Traditional Art of Baby Massage.* New York: Newmarket Press.

Lee, H.M., Kim, D.-H. and Yu, H.S. (2013) 'The effect of guided imagery on stress and fatigue in patients with thyroid cancer undergoing radioactive iodine therapy.' *Evidence-Based Complementary and Alternative Medicine.* Available at www.hindawi.com/journals/ecam/2013/130324/

Lepore, S.J., Buzaglo, J.S., Lieberman, M.A., Golant, M., Greener, J.R. and Davey, A. (2014) 'Comparing standard versus prosocial internet support groups for patients with breast cancer: A randomized controlled trial of the helper therapy principle.' *Journal of Clinical Oncology 32*, 36, 4081–4086.

Levy, L.M., Henkin R.I., Lin, C.S. Hutter, A. and Schellinger, D. (1999) 'Odor memory induces brain activation as measured by functional MRI.' *Journal of Computer Assisted Tomography 23*, 4, 487–498.

Lilius, J.M., Worline, M.C., Maitilis, S., Kanov, J., Dutton, J.A. and Frost, P. (2008) 'The contours and consequences of compassion at work.' *Journal of Organizational Behaviour 29*, 2, 193–218.

Looker, T.L. and Gregson, O. (1991) *Stresswise: A Practical Guide for Dealing with Stress.* London: Headway Books.

Luber, M. (2009) *Eye Movement Desensitization and Reprocessing, Scripted Protocols: Basics and Special Situations.* New York: Springer Publishing Co.

MacDonald, G. (2014) *Medicine Hands: Massage Therapy for People with Cancer.* Forres: Findhorn Press. [First edition 1999.]

McFarland, D. (1988) *Body Secrets: Unwinding Your Historical Limitations.* California: Healing Arts Press.

Mackereth, P.A. (2003) 'A minority report: Teaching fathers baby massage.' *Complementary Therapies in Nursing and Midwifery 9*, 3, 147–154.

Mackereth, P.A. and Carter, A. (eds) (2006) *Massage and Bodywork: Adapting Therapies for Cancer Care.* London: Elsevier.

Mackereth, P.A. and Dunn, K. (2017) 'Spirituality and Working Ethically at the End of Life.' In A. Carter and P.A. Mackereth (eds) *Aromatherapy, Massage and Relaxation in Cancer Care: An Integrative Resource for Practitioners* (pp.210–222). London: Singing Dragon.

Mackereth, P.A., Mehrez, M.J., Hackman, E. and Knowles, R. (2014) 'The value of complementary therapies for carers witnessing patients' medical procedures.' *Cancer Nursing Practice 13, 9, 32–38.*

Mackereth, P.A., Maycock, P., Mehrez, A. and Nightingale, L. (2016) 'Embedding a Palliative Care Therapy Service.' In A. Carter and P.A. Mackereth (eds) *Aromatherapy, Massage and Relaxation in Cancer Care: An Integrative Resource for Practitioners* (pp.89–105). London: Singing Dragon.

Marx, V. and Nagy, E. (2017) 'Fetal behavioral responses to the touch of the mother's abdomen: A frame-by-frame analysis.' *Infant Behavior and Development 47, 83–91.*

Maycock, P., Mackereth, P.A. and Carter, A. (2016) 'Aromasticks: A Portable Aromatic Powerhouse.' In A. Carter and P.A. Mackereth (eds) *Aromatherapy, Massage and Relaxation in Cancer Care: An Integrative Resource for Practitioners* (pp.118–129). London: Singing Dragon.

Menzies, V., Taylor, A.G. and Bourguignon, C. (2006) 'Effects of guided imagery on outcomes of pain, functional status, and self-efficacy in persons diagnosed with fibromyalgia.' *Journal of Alternative and Complementary Medicine 12, 1, 23–30.*

Monroe, K.R. (2002) 'Explicating Altruism.' In S.G. Post, L.G. Underwood, J.P. Schloss and W.B. Hurlbut (eds) *Altruism and Altruistic Love: Science, Philosophy and Religion in Dialogue (pp.106–122).* New York: Oxford University Press.

Montagu, A. (1986) *Touching: The Human Significance of the Skin* (3rd edn). New York: Harper & Row.

Moon, C.M. and Fifer, W.P. (2000) 'The fetus: Evidence of transnatal auditory learning.' *Journal of Perinatology 20, 8, Part 2, S37–S44.* Available at www.researchgate.net/publication/281313549

Morhenn, V., Beavin, L.E. and Zak, P.J. (2012) 'Massage increases oxytocin and reduces adrenocorticotropin hormone in humans.' *Alternative Therapies in Health and Medicine 18, 6, 11–18.*

National Cancer Institute (2018) 'SEER Training Modules.' Available at https://training.seer.cancer.gov

Nelson, A.M. (2017) 'Risks and benefits of swaddling healthy infants: An integrative review.' *MCN: American Journal of Maternal Child Nursing 42, 4, 216–225.*

Nelson, C.A. (2007) 'A neurobiological perspective on early human deprivation.' *Child Development Perspectives 1, 1, 13–18.*

NHS England (2014) *NHS Five Year Forward View.* Available at www.england. nhs.uk/five-year-forward-view/

O'Neil, P.M. and Calhoun, K.S. (1975) 'Sensory deficits and behavioral deterioration.' *Senescence: Journal of Abnormal Psychology 84, 579–582.*

Online Etymology Dictionary (2018) www.etymonline.com

Orlinsky, D.E., Grawe, K. and Parks, B.K. (1994) 'Process and Outcome in Psychotherapy.' In A.E. Bergin and S.I. Garfield (eds) *Handbook of Psychotherapy and Behaviour Change* (4th edn) (pp.270–376). New York: Wiley.

Patricolo, G.E., LaVoie, A., Slavin, B., Richards, N.L., Jagow, D. and Armstrong, K. (2017) 'Beneficial effects of guided imagery or clinical massage on status of patients in a progressive care unit.' *Critical Care Nurse 37*, 1, 62–69.

Penfield, W. and Boldrey, E. (1937) 'Somatic motor and sensory representation in the cerebral cortex of man as studied by electrical stimulation.' *Brain 60*, 389–440.

Polson, J. and Croy, S. (2015) 'Differentiating dementia, delirium and depression.' *Nursing Practice.* Available at www.nursingtimes.net/Journals/2015/04/10/v/n/b/150415_Differentiating-dementia-delirium-and-depression.pdf

Putz, R.V. and Tuppek, A. (1999) 'Evolution of the hand.' *Handchirurgie Mikrochirurgie Plastiscne Chirurgie 31*, 6, 357–361.

Rantala, J. (2017) 'The tactile senses and haptic perception.' Lecture 2. Tampere Unit for Computer-Human Interaction (TAUCHI), School of Information Sciences, University of Tampere, Finland. Available at www.uta.fi/sis/tie/hui/schedule/HUI2013-2-tactile-sensing.pdf

Rogers, C. (1951) *Client-centered Therapy: Its Current Practice, Implications and Theory.* London: Constable.

Rosetti, A., Chadha, M., Torres, B.N., Lee, J.K., Hylton, D., Loewy, J.V. and Harrison, L.B. (2017) 'The impact of music therapy on anxiety in cancer patients undergoing simulation for radiation therapy.' *International Journal of Radiation Oncology, Biology and Physics 1*, 99, 103–110.

Ross, M. (2000) 'Body talk: Somatic countertransference.' *Psychodynamic Counseling 6*, 4, 451–467.

Rothschild, B. (2004) 'Mirror, mirror: Our brains are hardwired for empathy.' *Somatic Trauma Therapy*, Sept/Oct. Available at www.somatictraumatherapy.com/mirror-mirror

Sabin-Farell, R. and Turpin, G. (2003) 'Vicarious traumatization: Implications for the mental health of health workers?' *Clinical Psychology Review 23*, 3, 449–480.

Sanderson, H., Harrison, H. and Price, S. (1991) *Aromatherapy and Massage for People with Learning Difficulties.* Birmingham: Hands On Publishing.

Satir, V. (1972) *Peoplemaking.* Mountain View, CA: Science and Behavior Books Inc.

Settle, F. (1991) 'My experience in a Romanian orphanage.' *Massage Therapy Journal*, Fall, 64–72.

Shahriari, M., Dehghan, M., Pahlavanzadeh, S. and Hazini, A. (2017) 'Effects of progressive muscle relaxation, guided imagery and deep diaphragmatic breathing on quality of life in elderly with breast or prostate cancer.' *Journal of Education and Health Promotion 19*, 6, 1.

Sinclair, S., Beamer, K., Hack, T.H. and McClement, S. (2017) 'Sympathy, empathy and compassion: A grounded theory study of palliative care patients' understanding, experiences and preferences.' *Palliative Medicine 31*, 5, 437–444.

Skedung, L., Arvidsson, M., Chung, J.Y., Stafford, C.M., Berglund, B. and Rutland, M.W. (2013) 'Feeling small: Exploring the tactile perception limits.' *Scientific Reports 3*. Available at www.ncbi.nlm.nih.gov/pubmed/24030568

Smith, E.W.L., Clance, P.R. and Imes, S. (1998) *Touch in Psychotherapy: Theory, Research, and Practice.* New York: Guilford Press.

Solomons, L., Solomons, J. and Gosney, M. (2013) 'Dementia and cancer: A review of the literature and current practice.' *Aging Health 9*, 3, 307–319.

Spratt, E.G., Back, S.E., Yeatts, S.D., Simpson, A.N., *et al.* (2009) 'Relationship between child abuse and adult smoking.' *International Journal of Psychiatry in Medicine 39*, 4, 417–426.

Stringer, J. and Donald, G. (2011) 'Aromasticks in cancer care: An innovation not to be sniffed at.' *Complementary Therapies in Clinical Practice 17*, 2, 116–121.

Subrahmanyam, K. and Greenfield, P. (2008) 'Online communication and adolescent relationships.' *The Future of Children 18*, 119–146.

Suzuki, M.T., Tatsumi, A., Otsuka, T., Kikuchi, K., *et al.* (2010) 'Effects of 6-week tactile touch intervention on elderly patients with dementia and nurses administering tactile touch.' *Alzheimer's & Dementia: The Journal of the Alzheimer's Association 25*, 8, 680–686.

Syrigos, K.N., Karachaliosis, D., Karapanangiotou, E.M., Nutting C.M., *et al.* (2009) 'Head and neck cancer in the elderly: An overview on the treatment modalities.' *Cancer Treatment Reviews 35*, 3, 237–245.

Tiran, D. and Mackereth, P.A. (2010) *Clinical Reflexology: A Guide for Integrated Practice.* London: Elsevier.

Upledger, J. (1997) *Your Inner Physician and You: CranioSacral Therapy and SomatoEmotional Release.* Berkeley, CA: North Atlantic Books.

Watson, M., Haviland, J.S., Davidson, J. and Bliss J.M. (1999) 'Influence of psychological response on survival in breast cancer: A population-based cohort study.' *Lancet 16*, 1331–1336.

Wilkinson, A.V., Barrera, S.L., McBride, C.M., Snyder, D.C., *et al.* (2012) 'Extant health behaviors and uptake of standardized vs. tailored health messages among cancer survivors enrolled in the FRESH START trial: A comparison of fighting-spirits vs. fatalists.' *Psycho-Oncology 21*, 1, 108–113.

FURTHER READING
AND ONLINE RESOURCES

FURTHER READING

The following books have been used either as resources for the development of the HEARTS Process or have been useful reference books. They are listed here as some of them are not well known, but they all have a place in a therapist's library.

The first 4 titles were the texts that had the most influence on the origins of The HEARTS Process. Other texts made a useful contribution as the different elements emerged.

Touch: An Exploration by Norman Autton (Darton, Longman & Todd, 1989): This is one of the foundation books for HEARTS. Although it was published in 1989, it covers the role of touch in society in detail from birth to death. It is an excellent read and copies are still available.

Touching: The Human Significance of the Skin by Ashley Montagu (Harper & Row, 3rd edn, 1986): This is another classic text. The content focuses on the skin and its role in tactile interaction in different cultures, and throughout all stages of human development. It is a substantial book – nearly 500 pages – and is another excellent read.

Body Secrets: Unwinding Your Historical Limitations by Don McFarland (Shi'Zen Publications, 2006; first published 1988): Although this is about massage, no physical techniques are described, and the text is more about the relationship between the therapist and 'the body' on which s/he is working and how the author perceives her/his work. The book offers a different dimension to body work, taking the reader into different perceptions of how we perceive the body and the person who is engaging in massage therapy.

Creative Imagery and Other Approaches to Healing by Rubin Battino (Crown House Publishing, 2000): If you love using guided imagery, it is likely that this book would be very useful. It is divided into two parts: Part One is about the principles, evidence, an analysis of scripts by well-known authors, placebo, methods and much more; Part Two is about psychotherapy-based approaches and is possibly more appropriate for counsellors and psychologists, although the content is still useful and interesting for complementary therapists.

Your Inner Physician and You: CranioSacral Therapy and SomatoEmotional Release by John Upledger (North Atlantic Books, 1997): A fascinating book about one of the gentlest of touch therapies. If you are interested in body work, the sensitivity of the hands and emotional release, this book would be of interest to you. Dr John Upledger takes you through the history and practice of craniosacral therapy using case histories and with references to body anatomy and physiology.

Bodywork – What Type of Massage to Get and How to Make the Most of It by Thomas Claire (Basic Health Publications, 2006): This book is for anyone who would like to explore other touch therapies apart from massage, reflexology and aromatherapy. It is somewhat subjective and anecdotal, as it is written from personal experience; however, there is much useful information about the therapies described in the book. Claire describes his experience of receiving 30 different therapies of bodywork, from shiatsu to rolfing, from polarity therapy to the Trager approach.

Medicine Hands: Massage Therapy for People with Cancer by Gayle MacDonald (Findhorn Press, 2014): This is a useful book for anyone who works with massage in cancer care. MacDonald describes the role of massage throughout treatment and during the recovery process. It is an evidence-based book that is well illustrated and contains good descriptions of clinical treatments and massage techniques supported by case histories.

Aromatherapy, Massage and Relaxation in Cancer Care: An Integrative Resource for Practitioners edited by Ann Carter and Peter Mackereth (Singing Dragon, 2017): This book has two sections – 'The Underlying Principles of Clinical Practice' and 'Practical Applications of Aromatherapy, Massage and Relaxation'. Its aim is to provide an evidence-based 'how to' book, so the first half is about the context of practice and the second half offers some practical applications of complementary therapies in clinical and supportive care settings.

The Compassionate Mind by Paul Gilbert (Constable and Robinson Ltd, 2013): Paul Gilbert is a professor at the University of Derby in the UK. He has written several books, and this one is particularly relevant to therapists as the content is about developing compassion for others and oneself. The first part of the book focuses on a theoretical approach that explores how our minds work and how compassion can become an antidote for stress. The second part includes practical tools for working with mindfulness, meditations and guided imagery, and is concerned with developing skills through exercises and worksheets.

NLP at Work: The Difference that Makes a Difference in Business by Sue Knight (Nicholas Brealey Publishing, 2002): This book is about using neuro linguistic processing (NLP) in the workplace. It has been included here as the explanations of NLP are clear and understandable. Although it is primarily a book for business, the text could easily be applied in a wide variety of settings.

ONLINE RESOURCES

The following list of websites supports mainly the content of Chapters 9 and 10. It is also intended as a resource list for readers who are seeking further information.

Admiral Nurses, specialist dementia nurses: www.dementiauk.org/ admiral-nurses

Age UK, the UK's largest charity working with older people: www. ageuk.org.uk

Alzheimer's Society, a care and research charity for people with dementia and their carers: www.alzheimersresearchuk.org

Cancer Research UK, for incidence, projections, disease, treatment options and patient information: www.cancerresearchuk.org/

Carers UK, a membership charity in the UK for carers: www. carersuk.org/forum

Dementia Friends, aiming to transform the way the nation thinks, acts and talks about dementia: www.dementiafriends.org.uk

Dementia UK, for sources of support for families, tips for communication and help sheets about getting a diagnosis of dementia: www.dementiauk.org and info@dementiauk.org

Lewy Body Society: www.lewybody.org

Macmillan Cancer Support Recovery Package: www.macmillan. org.uk/about-us/health-professionals/programmes-and-services/ recovery-package

National Institute for Health and Care Excellence (NICE), guidance for each tumour type and cancer services: www.nice.org.uk

National Institute on Aging (US): www.nia.nih.gov

Parkinson's UK: www.parkinsons.org.uk

INDEX